Motor Impairment
and
Compensatory Education

★ ★ ★

P. R. MORRIS

D.L.C., Dip.P.E.

Carnegie School of Physical Education,
City of Leeds and Carnegie College

AND

H. T. A. WHITING

M.A., Ph.D., D.L.C., A.B.Ps.S.

Department of Physical Education
Leeds University

LONDON: G. BELL & SONS LTD

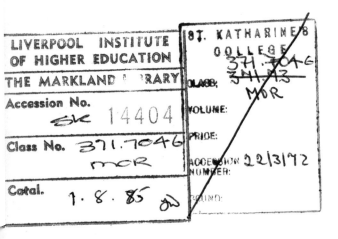
ISBN 0 7135 1802 2

Printed in Great Britain by
The Camelot Press Ltd, London and Southampton

Acknowledgements

We would like to express our gratitude to the following individuals for their help, guidance and provision of facilities in work carried out during the course of our investigations into the concept of motor impairment:

Dr. E. C. Allibone, Senior Lecturer in Paediatrics and Child Health, University of Leeds.
Mr. E. Bowskill, Senior Educational Psychologist, Leeds Child Guidance Centre.
Mr. J. B. Hill, Senior Remedial Teacher, Leeds Child Guidance Centre.
Mr. B. Hanwell, Headmaster, High Heath School, Sheffield.
Mr. G. D. Smith, Headmaster, St. Michael's School, Penkridge, Walsall.
Mr. R. Marks, Headmaster, Cardinal Square School, Leeds.
Mr. J. H. Taylor, Chief Education Officer, Leeds.
Mr. K. A. McClennan, Headmaster, and the staff of Cliff House School, Leeds.
Mr. R. W. Underwood, Headmaster ⎫ and the staff of Thorp Arch
Mr. W. L. Williams, Deputy Headmaster ⎬ Grange Junior Approved School.
Mr. Jones, Headmaster, and the staff of Rawmarsh Remedial Centre, Sheffield.

To the following students on the Diploma in Physical Education, Leeds University Institute of Education or the M.A. degree in Physical Education in the Department of Physical Education, University of Leeds, who provided so much of the source material and basic investigations:

Miss W. Allen, Miss J. Cooper, Mrs. A. Mumtaz and Messrs. G. J. K. Alderson, T. A. Clarke, J. G. Davies, P. J. Driver, P. E. Dyton, A. W. S. Garnett, I. M. Gibson, K. Hardman, G. F. Johnson, J. C. Jones, F. Luke, R. Lumley, B. Nettleton, M. Page, F. H. Sanderson, R. S. G. Sutcliffe, D. T. Voyce.

To the following authors, editors and publishers for permission to reproduce material from source texts:

6   MOTOR IMPAIRMENT AND COMPENSATORY EDUCATION

John Wiley & Sons., Inc., for permission to reproduce a table (Table 2) from Carmichael, J. (1952). *Manual of child psychology.* Messrs. Macmillan for permission to quote from Welton, J. (1912). *The psychology of education.* Charles E. Merrill Publishing Co., for permission to quote from Ismail, A. H. & Gruber, J. J. (1967). *Motor aptitude and intellectual performance.*

Fleishman, E. A. (1967). *Individual differences and motor learning.*

Benyon, S. D. (1968). *Intensive programming for slow learners.*

Indiana University Press for permission to quote from Osgood, C. E. & Sebeck, T. A. (Eds.) (1954). *Psycholinguistics.*

Charles C. Thomas publisher, Springfield, Illinois, and the author for permission to quote and reproduce a figure (Fig. 5) from Eysenck, H. J. (1967). *Biological basis of personality.*

Editors of Perceptual and Motor Skills and the authors for permission to reproduce a table (Table 4) from Sapir, S. G. & Wilson, B. M. (1967). *Patterns of developmental deficits. Percept. Motor Skills,* 24, 1291–1293.

Messrs. May & Baker and the author for permission to quote from Stott, D. H. (1962). Mongolism related to early shock in pregnancy. *Proceedings of the London Conference on the Scientific Study of Mental Deficiency.*

Mrs. J. R. Tamburrini for permission to quote from a paper presented at a conference in the School of Education, University of Sussex, 1968.

Editor of *Human Biology* for permission to reproduce a table (Table 1) from Hindley, C. B. *et al.* (1966). Differences in age of walking in five European longitudinal samples. *Human Biology,* 38, 4.

Editor *British Journal of Social and Clinical Psychology* for permission to reproduce a table (Table 5) from an article by Whiting, H. T. A. *et al.* (1969). The Gibson spiral maze as a possible screening device for minimal brain damage. *Brit. J. Soc. Clin. Psych.,* 8, 164–168.

Editor *Teacher Education in New Countries* for permission to reproduce a table from an article by Poole, H. (1969). Restructuring the perceptual world of African children.

Messrs. George, Allen & Unwin Ltd. for permission to quote from Gibson, J. J. (1966). *The senses considered as perceptual systems.*

Duke University Press for permission to quote from an article by Fisher, S. (1964). Body-awareness and selective memory for body versus non-body references. *J. Pers.,* 32, 138–144.

R. L. Underwood, headmaster of Thrope Arch School for permission to reproduce a poem by Neil Best.

Pergamon Press and the author for permission to quote from Meredith, G. P. (1966). *Instruments of communication.*

McGraw-Hill Book Co. for permission to quote from Farber, S. M. & Wilson, R. H. L. (Eds.) (1961). *Control of the mind.*

Editor *British Journal of Psychology* for permission to quote from Farmer, E. (1927). A group factor in sensory-motor tests. *Brit. J. Psych.,* 17, 4, 327–342.

British Psychological Society for permission to quote from Francis, R. D. (1968). A conative hypothesis. *Bull., Brit. Psych. Soc.*, 21, 241–244. Also for permission to reproduce Tables 1 and 2 from an article by Whiting, H. T. A., Clarke, T. A. and Morris, P. R. (1969). A clinical validation of the Stott Test of Motor Impairment. *Brit. J. Soc. Clin. Psych.*, 8, 270–274.

The College of Special Education for permission to quote from Frostig, M., in Arkwright, M. (1969). *The Frostig approach*.

The American Psychological Association for permission to quote from Lassner, R. (1948). Annotated Bibliography of the Oseretzky test of motor performance. *J. of Consult. Psych.*, 12, 37–47.

Harper and Row, publishers, for permission to quote from Gesell, A. and Amatruda, C. S. (1941). *Developmental diagnosis*.

Consulting Psychologists Press Inc., publishers, for permission to quote from *The developmental test of visual perception* by Marianne Frostig, Ph.D. (1966).

Editors of Developmental Medicine and Child Neurology, and Professor H. F. R. Prechtl for permission to quote from Prechtl, H. F. R. & Stemmer, C. J. (1962). The Chorieform syndrome in children. *Dev. Med. Child Neurol.* 4, 119–127, and the Editors for permission to quote from Stott, D. H. (1966). A general test of motor impairment for children. *Dev. Med. Child Neurol.*, 8, 523–531.

Editors of *Forward Trends* for permission to quote from Jakeman, D. (1967). The Marianne Frostig approach. *Forward Trends*, 11, 3, 99–110.

Grune and Stratton, publishers, and Laura Lehtinen for permission to quote from Strauss, A. A. & Lehtinen, L. (1948). *Psychopathology and education of the brain injured child*.

Editor of *Special Education* for permission to quote from Frostig, M. (1968). Sensory-motor development. *Special Education*, June, 18–20.

Editors of *The Lancet* for permission to quote from an article in volume 1 (1963), 1252.

Syracuse University Press for permission to quote from Cruickshank, W. M., Bentzen, F. A., Ratzeburg, F. H. and Tannhauser, M. T. (1961). *A teaching method for brain-injured and hyperactive children*.

The Williams & Wilkins Co., Baltimore, Md. 21202, U.S.A., for permission to quote from Spreen, O. & Benton, A. L. (1965). Comparative studies of some psychological tests of cerebral damage. *J. Nerv. Ment. Dis.* 5, 323–333, and for permission to quote from Fisher, M. (1956). Left hemiplegia and motor impersistence. *J. Nerv. Ment. Dis.*, 123, 201–218.

Editors of *Neurology* for permission to quote from Garfield, J. C. (1964). Motor impersistence in normal brain-damaged children. *Neurology*, 14, 623–630.

Editors of *Perceptual and Motor Skills* and the author for permission to quote from Espenschade, A. S. (1958). Kinesthetic awareness in motor learning. *Percept. Motor Skills*, 8, 142, and the Editors and the author for permission to quote from Vandenburg, S. G. (1964). Factor analytic study of the Lincoln/Oseretzky test of motor proficiency. *Percept. and Motor Skills*, 19, 23–41.

The Psychological Corporation for permission to quote and reproduce two tables (Table VII and IX) from Wechsler, D. (1949). *Wechsler intelligence scale for children*, Manual.

John H. Boydell, publisher, and the author for permission to quote Francis-Williams, J. (1964). Understanding and helping distractable children.

Professor W. Yule, Department of Child Development, University of London, for permission to quote from a paper presented at the Annual Conference of the British Psychological Society in April 1967, and for permission to quote from Yule, W., Graham, P. & Tizard, J. (1967) *Motor impersistence in 9-year-old children*. Unpublished paper.

Editors of Research Monographs for permission to quote from Bender, A. L. (1938). A visual-motor Gestalt Test. *Res. Monog.* 3, Amer. Orthopsychiatric Assn.

Editor of *Rehabilitation Literature* for permission to quote from Argy, W. P. (1965). Montessori versus orthodox. *Rehab. Lit.* 26, 10.

The Reading Research Foundation, Inc. for permission to quote from *Perceptual motor training* (1967).

The Minneapolis Educational Trust Bureau for permission to quote from Dell, E. A. (1946). *The Oseretzky tests of motor performance.*

Preface

This book represents the outcome of a number of years' work and lecturing on the topic of motor impairment to students on the advanced diploma course and M.A. degree in physical education at the University of Leeds. Work in this area was initially instituted as a counterbalance to the long-established interest amongst educationalists in the acquisition of high level skills.

To some extent, the inclusion of the term 'motor impairment' in the title can be misleading in that it suggests a limited focus of interest, whereas the subject matter of the book is much more far ranging, extending into a number of facets of education. While our primary concern is with manifested 'clumsy' behaviour, it would be wrong to infer that only the motor mechanisms are involved. This particular point is accordingly afforded detailed treatment in Chapter 1.

Motor impairment is seldom a unitary impairment. It has implications for skill acquisition in the social and intellectual field as well as the physical field. It would seem that in many cases a low level of ability to acquire skills in many areas may be present representing an impairment of a more general kind. A recognition of the interrelationship between the acquisition of social, intellectual and physical skills is reflected in the chapters specifically concerned with *motor impairment and the socialisation process* and *motor impairment and intellectual development*.

The term *compensatory education* is a comparatively new one and replaces to a large extent a former designation *re-education*. The latter term was often misused when standing for the former, since it implied educating once again people who had reached a particular educational level and who now for some reason did not exhibit behaviour (in the broadest sense) at a standard of which they were previously capable. Compensatory education on the other hand implies an attempt to make good a deficiency in a person's earlier education. While such a concept is understandable and a necessary one for the educationalist, it is open to question as to how successful such procedures are likely to be. A great deal of work has yet to be done on the innovation of methods designed to deal with the kinds of deficit which are becoming apparent. It is likely that traditional methods of approach to education are not suitable for compensatory education procedures. There is a need for well informed and imaginative teachers who can transcend the limitations imposed by stereotyped traditional procedures and the existing space/time frameworks of the present formal educational system. Although an attempt is made in Chapter 7 to bring together those compensatory education procedures which have been attempted by a few innovators in this field, it would appear that we are still some way from establishing a meaningful conceptual framework on which such procedures can be based.

The book is primarily designed as a source text for students of education and physical education in particular. It will no doubt in addition appeal to students of developmental psychology and workers in the field of child guidance and paediatrics. To this end, a deliberate attempt has been made to extend the source references to meet a variety of specific interests.

P. R. Morris
H. T. A. Whiting

Leeds
October 1970

Contents

Introduction

Motor impairment refers to the inadequacy of an individual's physical responses to the everyday demands of his environment. As such, it is a condition that manifests itself in performances which are subnormal or whose efficiency has been hampered in some way. These responses reflect inadequate attempts to perform those motor skills which can be regarded as being either essential or culturally desirable. In this context, the impairment signifies the inability of an individual to perform simple everyday tasks effectively in a controlled and coordinated manner.

The problem outlined

The consequences of this lack of ability constitute an educational problem, for there are many children both at school and of pre-school age who have difficulty in acquiring and performing even the simplest motor skills. The inadequacy of their responses may cause them to be labelled 'awkward' or 'clumsy'. This inability manifests itself particularly when such children are engaged in activities of a practical nature such as handicraft, painting, handwriting and games. At the pre-school and infant school level, they may have difficulty in using scissors, in constructing simple models, in manipulating objects and even in the everyday tasks of dressing and using a knife and fork.

The problem is further complicated by the fact that a motor-impaired child may be simultaneously a movement, an emotional, a neurological, an educational and a diagnostic problem. If an adequate compensatory education procedure is to be initiated and carried to fruition, integration of a number of concepts and research findings in the design of such a programme is necessary. Moreover, each impaired child must be considered not as simply belonging to a homogeneous category, but as an individual: his subnormal psycho-motor functioning must be viewed not as an isolated phenomenon, but as part of his total situation—his condition is the result of a mutually inclusive amalgam of physiological, environmental and interpersonal factors. Such an approach would lead to the construction of multi-dimensional profiles (Davitz *et al.*, 1964) of the individual, indicating—for example—his chronological age, motor ability, IQ, personality and the specific aetiology of his condition. If such profiles were available, predictions of typical course and outcome could be made with a greater degree of confidence.

Because of the multi-disciplinary involvement in the subject, there has been widespread, indiscriminate introduction of terminology from different theoretical standpoints sometimes resulting in fundamentally different definitions of similar entities. The need for a dominating theoretical framework providing sound and consistent terms of reference for researchers is frustrated by the seeming impossibility of the implementation of such an ideal in the present state of unsophisticated knowledge concerning aetiology, diagnosis and prognosis.

The specificity of motor impairment

Children who may be unable to perform a particular skill are not automatically incapable of acquiring other skills where different factors are involved. The hand-eye coordination of movements required to catch a ball may present difficulties to a child who, because of a visual defect, is unable to monitor the flight of the ball. On the other hand, the same child may be extremely proficient in throwing a ball to hit a stationary target. Some children who show a high degree of coordination and skill on the games field may have difficulty in performing the finer movements involved in handwriting.

It is also evident that, at the other end of the continuum, motor impairment may have far more global and far-reaching effects and limit a child's capability of performing and acquiring a wide variety of skills. In this case, when the cause is such as to produce severe impairment it seems probable that it may also be responsible for disturbances in other aspects of human performance. Fish (1961) for example noted that in children of school age, a derangement of motor and perceptual functions tended to be associated with an interference in intellectual functioning when the disturbance was sufficiently severe.

In order to determine the full meaning and extent of the problem, it is necessary to consider the manner in which these difficulties may affect children in respect of their education and normal development. Any generalisation as to the possible effects of motor impairment at this point, must be regarded as hypothesis rather than confirmed statements of fact. On this understanding, it is reasonable to suppose that a low standard of performance, coupled with the inability to perform certain simple tasks effectively, may result in a child having a limited vocabulary of motor skills and a correspondingly limited range of relevant experience upon which to base the development of abilities and the learning of further skills. This will inevitably lead to a slower rate of progress and a restriction in overall achievement and benefit. In extreme cases, there may be certain culturally desirable skills that some of these children never acquire, such as learning to sew or knit, or to produce legible handwriting. The syndrome therefore suggests that the children who are grossly impaired may have a limited potential in the acquisition of a wide range of skills.

Arising from these comments, one may justifiably hypothesise the possibility of other detrimental effects appearing as a by-product of the repeated lack of success and frustration during the learning process. In certain situations a child's lack of ability may bring him rebuke from the teacher or parent, and mockery from his classmates. He may be called 'lazy' or 'untidy' and even punished because of apparent carelessness, for when the cause of a child's difficulties is not obvious it is often assumed that there is no justifiable reason why his performance should be below that of any other child of the same age. By these reactions, a child is continually reminded that he is a failure yet little is done to counteract the psychological effects of his experience of failure.

It is conceivable that this form of intolerance from authority and from the peer group and the continual absence of recognition and personal prestige, may well have far-reaching and even damaging effects. Initially, there may be an immediate antipathy towards and avoidance of the particular activity and all that is associated with it. A possible consequence of this may be a restlessness and discontentment which becomes the prelude to social maladjustment or delinquent behaviour. Referring to this type of situation, in a study of thirty-three delinquent children in Glasgow, Stott (1966) has suggested that a motor-impaired child may compensate by alternative forms of achievement or assertion which are socially disapproved. In support of this, he found that there was a far greater incidence of motor impairment in the form of physical and neurological disturbances, including poor muscular coordination, in the delinquent children that he tested than in normal children.

In the absence of any substantial evidence there is only the suggestion of a relationship here, between the effects of repeated failure, avoidance behaviour and the search for alternative outlets and satisfactions which may lead to anti-social or even delinquent tendencies.

With the possibility of these wider implications, the full extent of the problem is extremely difficult to assess.

In a study by Brenner et al. (1967), which examined a sample of 810 children aged 8–9 years, 54 (6·7%) with IQ above 90 were regarded as being clumsy, in gait, in movement, or in fine motor control. Their school work had been constantly reported as untidy, careless and slovenly. The figure of 6·7% is a useful indication of the possible size of the problem in this instance. It is conceivable, that the percentage of children that are impaired may be considerably higher than this, particularly when the term impairment is considered as a problem in terms of the difficulties or lack of ability that some children may have in performing simple motor skills.

Even with the most valid and reliable measure it is impossible to impose a precise norm in order to identify the 'subnormal'. The placing of a 'cut-off' point is purely arbitrary for it is unrealistic to suggest that a single point on the scale can separate the performances of 'normal' children from those who by this criterion would be judged to be 'motor-impaired'. It is obvious that no clear division of this kind can be made for there exists a continuum of ability that ranges from the most proficient to the severely handicapped. While the extremes can be easily identified those who fall into the middle ranges are difficult to separate.

Today, a child would not necessarily be considered to be handicapped if he was for example unable to ride a bicycle, a skill that was more common only a few years ago. The necessity of a child to be able to tie his own shoe laces can now be avoided by providing him with the more convenient type of 'slip-on' shoes. The preponderance of new labour-saving devices makes life far less physically demanding both in terms of effort and skill.

A more liberal view of education has lessened the obligation made upon children to conform to prescribed patterns of skilled behaviour by allowing a more individual choice of action. Children are now encouraged to explore and find alternative ways of doing things within the accepted limitations of their own interests and abilities. Motor impairment has therefore become more generally accepted within the range of normality.

A child is now more able to ignore his weaknesses by avoiding many of the everyday tasks that confront him. If this can be done effectively, by adopting alternative measures that adequately meet the demands of the present situation, then the immediate problem ceases to exist. In this case, it is far more difficult to detect both the area and the cause of his weaknesses. Any manageable and efficient tests that would help to identify the children who are impaired in this way would do much to focus attention on their predicament and hence possibly allay any further damaging consequences. When these motor disabilities are recognised and accepted, then at the very least both teachers and parents may show a more sympathetic understanding and some form of compensatory education could be instigated in schools or medical treatment carried out for the more severe cases.

References

Brenner, M. W., Gillman, S. Zangwill, O. L. & Farrel, M. (1967) Visuo-motor ability in school children. *Brit. M. J.*, 4, 259–262.

Davitz, J. R., Davitz, L. J. & Lorge, I. (1964) *Terminology and concepts in mental retardation*. New York: Teachers College.

Fish, B. (1961) The study of motor development in infancy and its relation to psychological functioning. *Am. J. Psychiat.*, 17, 113–118.

Stott, D. H. (1966) A general test of motor-impairment for children. *Dev. Med. Child Neur.*, 8, 523–531.

CHAPTER 1

Motor Impairment—A Misnomer?

Skill is concerned with all the factors which go to make up a competent, expert, rapid and accurate performance.
(Welford, 1968)

The *description* of motor impairment used so far is in terms of skilled behaviour which has been adversely affected in some way and as a consequence is maladaptive. Such apparent emphasis on the output (effector/motor) side of performance is a natural one since it is this which makes its impact on the observer. Furthermore, it is with this manifested 'clumsy' behaviour that the parent, teacher or other member of society has to contend. The term *motor* impairment can, however, be a limitation when possible *explanations* of the deficiency in performance are being sought since this may give the impression that there is necessarily a deficit in the motor mechanisms themselves, whereas disturbances in one or more parts of a whole network of processes may be responsible for the observed *motor* impairment. Thus, it becomes necessary to adopt the more descriptive and acceptable term—perceptual-motor impairment. In so doing, attention is being drawn to the important relationship which exists between the input and output sides of performance. In some instances—such as cases of spasticity— the major fault may well lie with the effector mechanisms themselves, but with less well defined impairment, this may not necessarily be the case. For the remainder of this book, the reader should bear in mind that the term *motor impairment* will be used to imply a behavioural deficit in physical performance in a descriptive way and does not imply inferences about causality.

Model of perceptual-motor performance
The relationship which exists between the input and output

characteristics of skilled performance has been stressed by Argyle & Kendon (1967) in offering the following definition of skill:

> ... an organised, coordinated activity in relation to an object or a situation which involves a whole chain of sensory, central and motor mechanisms . . . the performance is continuously under the control of the sensory input . . . which controls the performance in the sense that outcomes of actions are continuously matched against some criterion of achievement or degree of approach to a goal according to which the performance is corrected.

Such a definition is sufficiently general as to embrace skills which are *primarily* motor as well as those which are *primarily* perceptual or *primarily* social.

In later chapters, the relationship between motor impairment and intellectual and social ability will be discussed. It is not inconceivable that where impairment in all three areas of performance occur together that they reflect a *general* underlying inability to acquire skill or a severely retarded *rate* of skill acquisition. The latter has been designated by McCloy (1954)— motor educability. Provins & Glencross (1968) have suggested that there appears to be a minimum level of general intelligence and motor capacity necessary for the acquisition of motor skill and that without these, handedness is also unable to develop.

To enable a better understanding of the mechanisms involved in perceptual-motor performance, it is useful to build up a model reflecting the major systems involved in such behaviour and to discuss the effect of damage, disturbance or failure to build up mediating processes at various parts of the model on the acquisition or performance of skilled acts. The description which follows reflects in the main concepts developed in the Cambridge School and in particular those of Welford (1968). A similar elaboration has been made by Whiting (1969) in relation to the acquisition and performance of ball skills. The model is an information processing one and while it has limitations which could be reduced by the application of statistical decision theory (Welford, 1968), it is considered to be useful in its present form within this context.

The gross physical systems which enter into the acquisition and performance of perceptual-motor skills are the sense organs, brain and muscles (Figure 1)

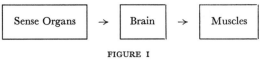

FIGURE I
Physical components

At a *functional* level, such physical components give rise to the reception of/or active seeking for input information via the sense organs or perceptual systems (Gibson, 1966), decision-making in the central mechanisms and output information via the muscles (Figure 2)

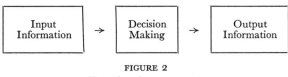

FIGURE 2
Functional components

Although much of the earlier work on skill concentrated on the input and output characteristics and their relationships (S–R psychology), it has become increasingly clear that it is necessary to postulate a further linking system between input and output reflecting the way in which decision making mediates between the input and output aspects of performance (S–O–R psychology). For this reason, the central mechanisms may be further elaborated in terms of the functions they are known to perform (Welford, 1968)—Figure 3. Thus, three primary subsystems are recognised—perceptual, translatory and effector.

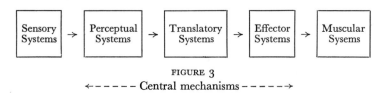

FIGURE 3
← – – – – – Central mechanisms – – – – – →

As a next stage in the development of the model and before further elaboration takes place, it is useful to combine these three simple models into a composite model with the addition of a feedback loop (one of very many within the system as a whole) between input and output (Figure 4).

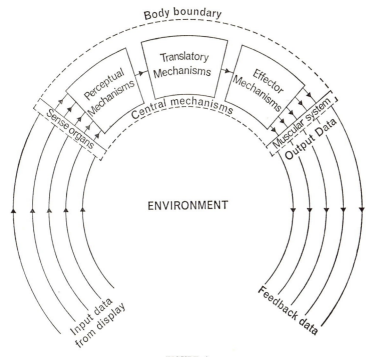

FIGURE 4

Model of perceptual-motor performance

While a model of this nature serves a useful purpose as an aid to understanding the extremely complex organisation involved in perceptual-motor performance, the reader should bear in mind the limitations which are imposed in attempting to depict dynamic processes in terms of a static model. While the overall systems depicted are probably correct, inside the 'black-boxes' is constant fluctuation, change and elaboration. The nervous system of the body is constantly active (in terms of the firing of nerve cells), the environment (both internal and external) is continually changing, attention fluctuates and man is never still. As Crossman (1964) has pointed out, adult skills are acquired piecemeal during a lengthy period of learning in childhood. The adult information system contains large amounts of stored information acquired through experience, serving to mediate in the performance of the subsystems and the system as a whole. Such information is continually being added to, modified and elaborated on the basis of further experience. The model must be conceived as dynamic.

At this stage of model building, it is instructive to elaborate on the general function of the system in perceptual-motor performance:

> Basically, in the performance of any perceptual-motor skill information from the display (immediate external environment in which the skill is to be carried out)—or about the internal environment (proprioceptive information) is relayed to the central mechanisms of the brain via the sense organs. Since the performer of a skill cannot utilise *all* the information available in the display at any one instant (because of limitations in his capacity to process information), *selective attention* determines both the area of the display which is scanned and the particular information which is abstracted. Sensory data from the external and internal environment is interpreted (the process of perception) in the central mechanisms on the basis of stored information acquired from past experience. On the basis of such perceptions, decisions are made with regard to new responses or adjustments to ongoing responses. If a response is to be made, the translatory mechanisms are responsible for linking the appropriate response patterns to such incoming information and the effector system gives the executive command to appropriate muscular systems. The carrying out of an effector response brings about a change in the display giving rise to 'feedback' information about the effectiveness of the response. Such information together with additional information from the display and the internal environment is available to be monitored by the sensory/perceptual systems and used in the control of ongoing behaviour or can be utilised in initiating and controlling future responses.

This brief outline has introduced a number of terms which may be of primary importance in elaborating the concept of motor impairment. Those which are considered to be of particular importance are developed further below.

Display

The display is that part of the external environment which contains information which is likely to be of use—or in some cases necessary—in the performance of the skill in question. It will be that part of the external environment towards which attention needs to be directed for the purpose of taking in information the processing of which will determine the appropriateness of the response. While in most instances information will be coming in via the visual system, and hence the display will refer to that 'which is before the performer's eyes' it must be remembered that in dealing with auditory information for example, the display may well be behind the skill performer. For this reason, Moray's (1969) use of the term 'input space' is perhaps more descriptive.

In many skilled performances, monitoring of the display plays a fundamental part in guiding the skilled behaviour while in others its importance may diminish as the performer becomes more competent. That is to say, that information from the external environment may play an important part in the learning of some skills but may become of less importance as skill develops. In many skills, there would appear to be a gradual changeover from the monitoring of external information to the monitoring of proprioceptive information and in some cases the pre-programming of the skill as a whole such that feedback information may play a very limited part in control. The problems involved in the changeover from visual to proprioceptive monitoring as skill develops have been discussed by Connolly (1969). He questions the ways in which a changeover from visual to proprioceptive analysers can be brought about.

Perception

In attempting to understand perception in relation to perceptual-motor performance, it is necessary to realise that the distance receptors (eyes and ears) which play such an important part in the monitoring of information from the environment are sensitive to incoming light or sound energy. At the receptors, the energy is converted into chains of electrical impulses (neural coding) and relayed to the central mechanisms via the appropriate nerves (Gregory, 1966).

Recently, Gibson (1968) has differentiated between passive receptors in terms of the sense organs themselves (e.g. retina of the eye) and the senses being considered as perceptual systems. When the senses *are* considered as perceptual systems, they actively seek out information from the environment. This implies an orientation of such perceptual systems (e.g. the eye,

eye in head, eye in head on body, etc.) towards particular parts of the display. Presumably, such orientation is the outcome of decision making in the central mechanisms brought about by specific directions to the musculature and can itself be considered as an example of skilled behaviour. It is also possible that a particular stimulus subset from the display may itself result in the orientation of the sense organs without the mediation of the central mechanisms such as occurs when stimulation at the extreme edge of the retina initiates a reflex which causes the eye to rotate bringing the moving object into central vision.

Sensory information impinging on the receptors gives rise to the patterns of brain activity the processing and interpretation (on the basis of past experience) of which constitutes the act of perception.

Selective attention

One aspect of this procedure has already been elaborated in relation to the perceptual systems actively seeking out information. Because of the limitations of the sense organs, the amount of information present in the display, the need to orientate the perceptual systems to particular parts of the environment and the necessity for information to be obtained with an optimum level of speed and accuracy it is necessary for attention to be selective. By this is meant that either consciously or unconsciously, attention is focused on a particular part of the display. The patterns of fixation are themselves skilled acts—partly pre-planned but also using feedback so adjusted that the average rate of intake of information remains within the capacity of the later processing systems. The criterion of success in terms of selective attention is the ability to extract the information necessary for making the skilled behaviour adaptive. It will be appreciated in this respect, that one of the requirements of a good teacher of skills is that he knows what information within a display is worth attending to, i.e. those particular stimulus subsets which give rise to information the monitoring of which is essential for the performance of the skill at a particular level. It appears that stimuli which are not attended to are excluded from perception (Horn, 1966) so that a person may also be considered to demonstrate selective *perception*. It is also worth noting, that in concentrating attention on relevant stimuli, it is necessary to ignore stimuli which are irrelevant. As Rabbitt (1967) has pointed out, this may equally well be a learned ability.

As well as selective attention to particular aspects of the display in terms of the orientation of the perceptual systems, it is necessary to consider further the mechanisms which exist for ensuring that the brain itself is not continuously bombarded by diffuse sensory input much of which may carry redundant information. This topic will be dealt with under the heading of *filtering*.

Feedback

Although feedback is a common enough term in relation to the control of machine systems, its adoption in the description of human control systems is comparatively recent and would appear to have developed from Wiener's (1948) elaboration of Cybernetics (the science of control and communication). Although the analogy between the control of machine-systems and the control of the human system is a useful one, there are important differences in the characteristics of the two systems (Milhorn, 1966). In terms of the human control system, feedback is often designated 'knowledge of results'. Holding (1966) with others distinguishes between internal and external feedback. Internal feedback—in terms of proprioceptive information—is intrinsic to all human performance. External feedback—represented by changes in the display—may be intrinsic to a particular performance in as far as it is the direct result of the action. However, it may also be provided by an external agency (such as a teacher) giving rise to what has been termed *augmented knowledge of results*.

Armed with these basic concepts, it is now necessary to elaborate the model still further in order to account for further subsystems in which damage, disturbances or failures in development may lead to a breakdown in skilled performance and manifest motor impairment.

Filtering

To stress the point which was made under the heading of selective attention, it is clear that the nervous system of man has a limited capacity for processing information (Welford, 1968). In addition, the processing of unnecessary (to the task in hand) information may lead to delays in decision making necessary for adaptation. For this reason, the diverse stimulation impinging on the sensory receptors needs to be filtered. There are two further main reasons why this should be necessary:

1. So that the information processed is that which makes subsequent behaviour adaptive.
2. Prevention of overactivation of sensory neurons in the cortex and therefore an excessive bombardment of the brain by afferent impulses.

The point being made in 2. will be developed further under the heading of *Arousal*.

The question now, is how specific information is selected from the sensory input and how such selection is influenced by prior experience. One way of course is by the orientation of the perceptual systems previously discussed. This in itself is not sufficient as even when orientation is achieved, the amount of potential stimulation falling on the sensory receptors is still large. From the developing work in this area, it would appear that central nervous system processes determined by memories, emotional states (which may reflect genetic predispositions), etc., can facilitate or inhibit sensory input patterns by means of systems of fibres that run from the brain to synaptic regions in the afferent pathways (Livingston, 1959; Melzack, 1968). These may not be the only filter mechanisms. Marler (1961) for example has proposed three types of filtering system:

1. That imposed primarily by the receptors (on the basis of their physical structure or biases which have been imposed by facilitatory or inhibitory feedback mechanisms from the C.N.S.).
2. By the receptor afferent pathways and the C.N.S. as they function together in normal perception.
3. By a central filtering mechanism.

Welford (1968) has, however, argued that experimental findings may be capable of interpretation in terms of *one* filter system in the perceptual mechanisms. The difficulties in this field and the differences of opinion which exist have been discussed by Treisman (1969) and Moray (1969).

The concept of sensory and perceptual filtering is not a new one. Major developments in this area would appear to have been brought about by the work of Broadbent (1956). His earlier work led him to postulate a filter mechanism between the sense organs and the central mechanisms which would allow only signals with particular physical characteristics or from particular sense organs to be relayed further. Developing work in the area suggests that an interpretation of this nature is too simple, the implication being that a purely peripheral interpretation is insufficient and that there must be some analysis of the data before particular information is relayed further.

To summarise, it would seem necessary from the experimental evidence to postulate a filter mechanism(s) to account for some of the characteristics of selective attention and that at the present state of knowledge such a filter system(s) may be peripheral, central or part of both systems. The overlap which exists between the concepts used by different workers to account for such mediating mechanisms are of interest. Thus, Piaget (1950) speaks of 'schemata', Deutsch (1960) and Sutherland (1959) of 'analysers', Mackay (1962) of 'comparators' and Broadbent (1956) and Treisman (1969) of 'filter mechanisms'. It is also likely that Fleishman's (1967) concept of 'abilities' in terms of information processing potential may be similarly related.

Arousal

If processes of facilitation and inhibition affect the amount and kind of stimulation getting through to the cortex from the sensory receptors and from the cortex to the muscular systems, what sort of mechanisms are postulated for this purpose? Summarising a large number of recent neurological studies, Samuels (1959) concludes that all sensory modalities both interoceptive and exteroceptive give off collaterals to both the brain stem and the thalamic reticular systems (Figure 5). Thus, visual, auditory, olfactory, tactile, pain, proprioceptive and visceral stimuli are all capable of activating both components of the reticular formation.

The reticular formation comprises nerve cells scattered throughout the brain stem. The thalamic reticular system is sometimes designated the visceral brain and is responsible for control and activation of the autonomic nervous system. It is to the reticular system that has been ascribed the facilitatory and inhibitory functions related to filtering that have been previously mentioned.

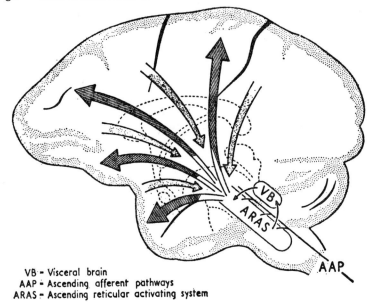

VB - Visceral brain
AAP - Ascending afferent pathways
ARAS - Ascending reticular activating system

FIGURE 5
Brain-stem and thalamic reticular systems   (from Eysenck 1967)

It must also be remembered that incoming sensory stimulation is not projected on to an inert and inactive cortex. The cortical system is always to some degree *activated* or *aroused* (tonic arousal). While in many cases the latter two terms are used synonymously, Eysenck (1967) elaborates on these as follows:

> We have two sets of loops which are in turn connected with each other. The first of these is the cortico-reticular loop. Neural messages going along the classical ascending afferent pathways relay to the particular projection areas involved in the cortex; they also send collaterals into the reticular formation which in turn sends 'arousal' messages to the cortex to keep it in a state of functional tonus. Depending on the nature of the information transmitted the cortex in turn instructs the reticular formation to continue sending arousal messages or else to switch to inhibition. This loop then is concerned with information processing with cortical arousal and inhibition and in its application to personality differences with introversion and extraversion.

Although there is some degree of partial independence between autonomic activation and cortical arousal, activation always leads to arousal but arousal very frequently arises from types of stimulation which do not involve activation.

Much of the literature concern so far has been with the effect of the reticular formation on afferent stimulation, it would appear that it also has a direct facilitatory or inhibitory effect on motor outflow.

There would appear to be an optimal level of arousal which best facilitates performance. This is reflected in the Yerkes–Dodson law (recently revived by Broadhurst (1959)) which briefly proposes that:

> . . . an easy discrimination is more easily learned by an animal the higher the motivation but that for more difficult discriminations learning is best at an intermediate level of motivation, the optimum value shifting to a lower level as the discrimination becomes harder. (Broadbent 1965)

Eysenck (1967) has also proposed that the optimal level is higher for persons towards the extraverted end of the introversion/extraversion continuum.

Memory

Memory is concerned with the retention of information in the central mechanisms over a period of time. When the time is short—a matter of seconds—the label short-term memory is used.

In learning to perform skills, it has been pointed out that it is necessary to take in information from the environment over a period of time. Such information is retained in short-term memory initially and used to guide the performance of the skill. This is particularly the case when a person is required to 'imitate' the actions of a particular model. In the case of information held in a short-term memory store, the difficulty may lie purely in the limitation of such a store. Motor-impaired children are often found to have a deficiency in this mechanism. In being asked to reproduce objects from memory, it would be expected in such instances that the latter part of the reproduction would deteriorate as the memory faded. This is not necessarily so, as the learner is likely to rehearse the image verbally to prevent decay. Again, the first part of the figure might give clues to fire-off long-term memory of such figures. Related to this aspect of disturbance is the likely possibility that in being asked to imitate or draw from memory a particular aspect of the environment, the learner instead of retaining a representational image, verbalises the object to be reproduced. A disturbance in the form of an inadequate conceptual framework could limit the learner's ability in this respect leading to the reproduction of a wrong model but not it should be noted because the learner is incapable of performing the primarily motor skill involved in the reproduction.

A deficiency in the permanent memory store can lead to inadequate filtering of inputs because of a failure to appreciate the significance of stimuli. Such significance would normally be built up by satisfactory early experience. In such cases, Melzack (1968) suggests that the total input bombarding the C.N.S. produces an excessive arousal which as Hebb (1955) has suggested could be responsible for the correspondingly low cue properties necessary for discrimination and adaptive response.

Application of the Model

While the composite model outlined serves the useful purpose of focusing attention on the diverse subsystems involved in any skilled performance, it also makes explicit the numerous disturbances which can affect the functioning of such subsystems or prevent the building up of mediating processes vital to adaptive behaviour. Physical damage to the brain can upset the functioning of particular subsystems and in the developing organism can affect the building up of such mediating systems. In addition, a failure to establish the correct linkages and feedback mechanisms between subsystems can lead to inefficient functioning. Temporary disturbances may also play their part in causing temporary decrements in performance which could be misinterpreted if observation of a particular case of motor impairment were for example restricted to one occasion. In this respect, it is instructive to note the work of Schaffer & Emerson (1968) who showed the effect on developmental quotient test performance when young children were deprived of normal stimulation for a period of hours prior to the testing procedure. Such children showed a marked fall-off in developmental quotient compared with that achieved under conditions of normal stimulation.

To give more explicit examples of the way in which poor

skill performance should be related to various parts of the model, it is worth elaborating some hypothetical considerations. Assuming for example that the skill to be performed requires the taking in of information from the display for its correct performance, a number of disturbances may affect the ability of the performer to do so adequately. In the first place, the performer may fail to orientate himself towards that part of the display where necessary information can be found. This may be due to lack of experience in similar situations, i.e. to a failure in the conceptual framework of the memory store or a failure on the part of the filter systems to extract the relevant information from the totality impinging on the perceptual systems. In part, this could imply a defect in the receptors themselves and certainly such systems should form part of any initial check.

It is possible for the learner to focus his attention on the right part of the display from which the relevant information is available, but to put a wrong interpretation on the sensory input selected—a failure in the perceptual mechanisms influenced by memory stores. This is most clearly shown in the presence of well-known illusions, but it would seem likely that it is more generally applicable. Another interpretation in this case might be the inaccessibility of the memory trace. That is to say, that the learner has experienced the situation previously and has stored data to that effect but is unable to call it up at the right time—either because it is literally inaccessible or because the time taken to recall makes it no longer applicable to the particular situation.

To push the example on further. The subject may orientate himself in the right direction, select and put the correct interpretation on the incoming sensory input but make a wrong translation. That is to say that he makes an inappropriate response. Reasons for this may again rest with limited experience resulting in a failure to build-up stimulus-response compatabilities. Again, the procedure may be carried out effectively even up to the correct translation but the muscular system may be incapable of carrying out the directions of the effector mechanisms.

It is unlikely that the hypothetical situations described do in fact exist in such a clear-cut way. What seems more probable, is that a failure in any one part of the system will affect the development of other parts. That is to say, that a reciprocal relationship probably exists between the various subsystems such that gross disturbances at least will lead to a lowered capacity for acquiring skill of any kind.

The problems raised in this section will become more meaningful when the aetiology of motor impairment is elaborated in the next chapter.

References

Argyle, M. & Kendon, A. (1967)   The experimental analysis of social performance. In L. Berkowitz (Ed.) *Advances in experimental social psychology*, Vol. 3. New York: Academic Press.

Broadbent, D. E. (1956)   *Perception and communication*. London: Pergamon.

Broadbent, D. E. (1965)   A reformulation of the Yerkes–Dodson Law. *Brit. J. Math. Stat. Psych.*, 18, 2, 145–157.

Broadhurst, P. L. (1959)   The interaction of task difficulty and maturation: the Yerkes–Dodson Law revived. *Acta Psychologica*, 16, 321–338.

Connolly, K. (1969)   The applications of operant conditioning to the measurement and development of motor skill in children. *Dev. Med. & Child Neur.*, 10, 6, 697–705.

Crossman, E. R. F. W. (1964)   Information processes in human skill. *Brit. Med. Bull.* 20, 1, 32–37.

Deutsch, J. A. (1960)   *The structural basis of behaviour*. London: Cambridge Universtiy Press.

Eysenck, H. J. (1967)   *The biological basis of personality*. Springfield: Thomas.

Fleishman, E. A. (1967)   Individual differences and motor learning. In R. M. Gagne (Ed.) *Learning and individual differences*. Ohio: Merrill.

Gibson, J. J. (1968)   *The senses considered as perceptual systems*. London: George, Allen & Unwin.

Gregory, R. L. (1966)   *Eye and Brain*. London: Unwin.

Hebb, D. O. (1955)   Drives and the C.N.S. *Psych. Rev.* 62, 243–254.

Holding, D. H. (1966)   *Principles of training*. London: Pergamon.

Horn, G. (1966)   Physiological and psychological aspects of selective perception. In D. S. Lehrman, R. A. Hinde & E. Shaw (Eds.) *Advances in the study of behaviour*. New York: Academic Press.

Livingston, R. B. (1959)   Central control of receptors and sensory transmission systems. In J. Field (Ed.) *Handbook of physiology.* Section 1: Vol. 2. Washington: Amer. Physiol. Soc.

Mackay, D. M. (1962) Theoretical models of space perception. In C. A. Muses (Ed.) *Aspects of the theory of artificial intelligence.* New York: Plenum.

Marler, P. (1961) The filtering of external stimuli during instinctive behaviour. In W. H. Thorpe & O. L. Zangwill (Eds.) *Current problems in animal behaviour.* London: Cambridge University Press.

McCloy, C. H. (1954) *Tests and measurements in health and physical education.* New York: Crofts.

Melzack, R. (1968) A neuropsychological approach to heredity environment. In M. G. Newton & S. Levine (Eds.) *Early experience and behaviour.* Springfield: Thomas.

Milhorn, H. T. (1966) *The application of control theory to physiological systems.* London: Saunders.

Moray, N. (1969) *Attention.* London: Hutchinson.

Piaget, J. (1950) *The psychology of intelligence.* London: Routledge & Kegan Paul.

Provins, K. A. & Glencross, D. J. (1968) Handwriting, typewriting and handedness. *Q.J. Exp. Psych.,* XX, 3, 282–289.

Rabbitt, P. M. (1967) Learning to ignore irrelevant information. *Am. J. Psych.,* 80, 1, 1–13.

Samuels, I. (1959) Reticular mechanisms and behaviour. *Psych. Bull.,* 56, 1–25.

Schaffer, H. R. & Emerson, P. E. (1968) The effects of experimentally administered stimulation on developmental quotients of infants. *Brit. J.Soc. Clin. Psych.,* 7, 61–67.

Sutherland, N. S. (1959) *Stimulus analysing mechanisms.* In Proceedings of a symposium on the mechanisation of thought processes. Vol. 2. London: H.M.S.O.

Treisman, A. M. (1969) Strategies and models of selective attention. *Psych. Rev.,* 76, 3, 282–299.

Welford, A. T. (1968) *Fundamentals of skill.* London: Methuen.

Whiting, H. T. A. (1969) *Acquiring ball skill*—a psychological interpretation. London: Bell.

Wiener, N. (1948) *Cybernetics.* New York: Wiley.

CHAPTER 2

Aetiology of Motor Impairment

Children are conceived, born and grow—the products of nurturing ingredients of life, love, acceptance and parental devotion. Introduce a disturbance—of conception (congenital defect), of birth (brain damage) or of growth (personality disturbance)—and more of these nurturing ingredients are needed. Combine some of these disturbances and an extra-ordinary nurturing effort is required, effort which is not, unfortunately, always made. Too often the defect, damage or disturbance breeds anxiety, rejection, isolation—and further disturbance. And so a destructive cycle is initiated.

(Donague & Nichtern, 1965)

This quotation makes explicit the aetiological problem of motor impairment. In the previous chapter care was taken to emphasise the fact that any skilled behaviour involves a whole network of subsystems which acting together as an integrated whole contribute to efficient performance.

At an everyday level, a child who is considered to be motor-impaired is observed to be unable to perform the particular patterns of skilled behaviour demanded by his environment. Not only is his performance below the norm, but it is sufficiently poor as to make his behaviour in general or in specific situations maladaptive. If this were not so, the problem would be less obvious. Such patterns of skilled behaviour are determined by cultural factors as well as by age, sex, level of maturation and the environmental background of the child concerned. This in itself can lead to a failure to appreciate the likely magnitude of the problem. If the immediate situation does not make many demands on the child (for example if someone else ties up his shoes or dresses him) his inability may go unnoticed. In a more sophisticated environment and particularly one containing children of reasonably high skilled ability a child might be considered to be impaired when his standard of performance would be not unusual in a less sophisticated environment. The child who is deemed impaired in a poor environmental setting (e.g. amongst children of low skill ability) would appear to be *extremely* impaired if his environment changed for some reason to a more sophisticated setting.

The true magnitude of the problem of motor impairment and the way in which it relates to or is even a causal factor in other areas of impairment (verbal, social, emotional) will not be appreciated until tests exist which are universally valid. The problems and difficulties of test construction are discussed in a later chapter.

In a sense, therefore, the problem of motor impairment is one that has been created by the demands made upon the individual to learn certain skills that are regarded as important or at least desirable from a normal developmental viewpoint. It is perhaps significant that few children can avoid the necessity (from an acceptance point of view) of learning quite sophisticated motor skills in the course of their everyday play activities with other children. Seldom does the physically adept child encounter difficulties of social integration. If the child is not observed to show a deficiency in the performance of everyday tasks within the home, school or play, environment deterioration in other aspects of his development might be wrongly interpreted. It is perhaps the educated parents who are first to notice an impaired performance in their child. The fact that a problem does exist and that it is recognised as such by many parents is illustrated by the following extracts from letters which were received in response to press publicity on motor impairment:

My son, eleven years of age, has very poor coordination. This was first noticed when he was learning to walk which he began to do about 10 and a half months of age. He was unsteady in balancing himself. As he grew older we noticed that he stumbled frequently, and in fighting with other boys, his punches never seemed to land where he aimed. This has been a definite handicap to him because since he is poor in defending himself he is constantly on the defensive. Athletically he is 'scorned' by boys his own age. This has also been a handicap. He suffers socially with children who are aware of his handicap. Intellectually he is very bright. He is a good reader and reasons well.

We have been advised by one doctor, the only one to whom we have spoken that apparently(?) there is a very mild brain damage and since there is nothing able to be done, we must not let him know that he has this damage. I have always felt that there must be something that we can do.

Perhaps it is too late psychologically to help my child because the scars of ridicule by other children and his own awareness of his lack of ability and my own over-protectiveness might be too deep.

When ———— went into the first grade, this past September, his teacher said she was completely puzzled. I went in for his test results on evaluation in November and she asked me why he was so unsteady in physical education, drawing, holding a pencil, things of that sort. I told her he had been that unsteady type since birth and that he was so much better now than he had been at three and four years of age. I said, 'Personally, I feel children are born this way and it is a handicap.' She almost laughed in my face. She also said that on first evaluation they thought my child was 'slow' but found out that he was very bright and not an average child at all mentally. They tested him (all of the children were tested) on the basis of a 3% equivalency or third grade comprehension in reading and understanding and his tests came out a 2·5%. The class average ran a 1·4%. He was given a straight '1' on everything requiring understanding such as mixing-matching tests, phonics, science, maths., reading and sentence structure but he was given 3's on subjects requiring adroitness or agility. These were physical education, drawing, water coloring, playing ball, etc. This nearly crushed the child as he is a sensitive type and gets upset when he knows he is doing something poorly or in an awkward manner.

He has lost two of his neighborhood buddies because he can't play ball well enough to suit them and that is all they want to do. The fact that he does better than they in school doesn't seem to console him when he wants to play.

This account would seem to describe my son who is 5½ years old. His poor coordination has affected him socially for at least the last two years. A year ago, I took him for a check-up at the local cerebral palsy clinic which is all there is available in this area. The doctor didn't even examine him and only casually watched him walk in and then said he was perfectly normal in all respects.

Granted he is within 'normal' limits! However, there has always been 'something slightly off'. He falls constantly without being aware of why—small muscle coordination is poor—it's difficult for him to hold a pencil.

His background leaves a possible chance for birth injury. He was $7\frac{1}{2}$ weeks premature and was born within 20 minutes after the amniotic sac burst—fast and furious. He weighed in at 4 pounds 13 ozs. and lost to a 3 pounds 14 ozs. He was slightly hyperactive and remained in the incubator at the hospital for one month when he was discharged weighing 5 pounds 2 ozs. This was my first pregnancy.

A deficiency in skilled behaviour on the part of a person may be the result of:

(a) A *breakdown* in already established skill ability.
(b) An inherent inability to carry out successfully the skill which is demanded of him.

In talking about a *breakdown* in skilled performance, the implication is that the person is now unable to perform a skilled act(s) where previously such an ability had existed. This may be temporary or permanent. The breakdown may be due to physical damage to the brain itself or some toxic influence such as might be experienced by the drug-addict or alcoholic. Again, such damage may result in immediate impaired performance or may accumulate with time finally bringing about a noticeable impairment. In the main, interest in this chapter will not centre around difficulties of this kind since the antecedent conditions (unless long protracted) will generally be appreciated and the diagnosis more obvious. However, such conditions and possibilities should certainly be borne in mind by anyone concerned with the diagnosis and compensatory education of motor impaired children.

The second sense in which motor impairment has been used will be the major concern of this chapter. That is to say, that the concern will be with the child who has never acquired the ability to perform particular skilled acts demanded of him rather than that he once had the ability and now for some reason has lost this ability. A two-fold distinction is worth making in respect to such children:

1. The child is *backward* in terms of motor ability. That is to say his present ability does not match his potential at this stage of development. There might be a large number of reasons why this should be so, and it also begs the question of assessment of potential.

2. The child is a slow learner in the sense that his potential *rate* of development is far below that of the normal child of the same age. He is in no sense *backward* since his rate of development is all that might be expected.

In either of these cases, the difficulty of attributing the deficit to particular causal factors is apparent. Primarily, consideration must centre around genetic predisposition, brain damage, or an impoverished environment (in the sense of a lack of opportunity to experience in a specific or in a more general way). Such causal factors are not necessarily isolated and interactions between some or all of these are to be expected. The brain-damaged child for example would be more likely to suffer from the effects of deprivation. Genetic predisposition of the mother or child might determine the possibility of brain damage in the developing foetus. The possibility and more likely the probability of multi-determination of impairment with little likelihood of being really specific must not be overlooked. These are the kind of problems which are likely to face any person concerned with compensatory education.

It is considered useful here, to avoid some of the problems posed by a consideration of the integrated effects of genetic predisposition, brain damage and environmental deprivation by looking at the latter two areas separately and commenting on the former where appropriate.

To some extent, consideration of such causal factors can lead to an infinite regress in as far as it is being said that the reason(s) for the observed impairment are a, b, c, etc. It must then be asked, what are the reasons for the presence of a, b, c, etc.? Nevertheless, there comes a time at which a particular level of analysis will be more appropriate to those concerned with preventative medicine in both a physical and social sense rather than those people dealing with the problem as it exists, i.e. concerned with compensatory education.

Brain damage
The impaired perceptual-motor performances so often linked

with *known* cases of brain damage have in the past led investigators to generalise to other instances of perceptual-motor impairment where brain damage is less apparent. This is not altogether surprising since observation of behavioural deficits in perceptual-motor functioning is one of the earliest signs that something may be wrong. A brain-damaged child might be expected to show disturbances in some or all of the following—perception, concept formation, emotional and social development and in motor performance—depending upon the seat of the damage, and the stage in development at which it occurred. Perceptual and conceptual deviations have also been associated with distractibility, perseveration and disinhibition together with associated disturbances in visual, auditory and tactile functioning.

Brain damage *per se* gives the impression of a structural change brought about by physical causes, toxic reactions and anoxia. These are certainly of importance and will be discussed below. However, a failure to detect signs of organic damage does not necessarily imply the absence of what has been termed *brain dysfunction*. While such a concept may have mentalistic overtones and thus be unacceptable to some readers and considered by others to be a term which covers a multitude of sins, it does at least widen the field of consideration. This possibility will be discussed more fully later in the chapter.

How general is the concept of brain damage? Knobloch & Pasamanick (1959a) have postulated a continuum of reproductive casualty extending from foetal deaths (abortions, stillbirths and neonatal deaths) through a descending gradient of brain damage manifested in cerebral palsy, epilepsy, mental deficiency and behaviour disorders in childhood. Such deficiencies are particularly associated with maternal complications during pregnancy all of which can lead to foetal anoxia. Support for such a continuum comes from the work of Lilienfeld, *et al.* (1955) and Rogers *et al.* (1955). More recently, Corah *et al.* (1965) in reporting on a longitudinal study into the effects of perinatal anoxia after an interval of seven years showed that the anoxic groups suffered impairment in the areas of verbal abstract ability, perceptual skill and social competence. These workers, however, suggest that attempts to predict current functioning from newborn measures of severity of anoxia are highly unreliable.

On the basis of the Knobloch & Pasamanick continuum, we are all brain damaged and it is simply a matter of degree! The problem then reduces to the interactive effects of greater or lesser damage with environmental opportunity.

Such a concept of brain damage should not be overlooked. Depending upon the severity and location, the damage may have the effect of reducing the original (at conception) potential of the child and of changing both the manner and the means by which a child may reach his new potential. It also implies that there is a quantitative difference in the associated behavioural abnormalities throughout this range. It is significant therefore that at the minimal level a child who has brain damage may be more physically competent than one who has for example suffered through an unfavourable environment.

A concept of this nature may also influence the way in which compensatory education procedures are organised and in addition, acceptance of the existence of such a continuum may lead to concern about the prevention of such damage particularly directed towards a consideration of inter-uterine development and birth injuries. Stott (1957) for example has drawn attention to the effects of 'stress' during pregnancy on the developing foetus and Heyns (1963) has developed a system of abdominal decompression aimed at the prevention of foetal anoxia (see, however, critique of Liddicoat, 1968).

According to Strauss & Kephart (1955) the possible causes of brain damage, pre, para and postnatal are premature birth, caesarean sections, dry births, precipitate deliveries, eclampsia, pelvic malformations, antepartum haemorrhage, anomalies in presentation, twisting of the umbilical cord, use of forceps, improper use of anaesthetics, placenta praevia, rhesus incompatability, hereditary defects and hormone disturbance.

These factors have been classified by Caldwell (1956) into four groups:

Prenatal	(1)	defects in germ plasm
	(2)	deleterious influences of noxious agents affecting the embryo, foetus and infant
Paranatal	(3)	birth injuries of all types, chemical and mechanical (presentation anomalies and cephalo-pelvic disproportion)
Postnatal	(4)	postnatal infection or insult.

and will be discussed under these sub-headings:

Prenatal effects

Prenatal factors causing congenital malformations may act at any time from conception to the onset of labour. Such malformations are said to account for 30% of brain injuries. Of ninety-five children with congenital defects studied by Murphy (1948) 60% had anomalies of the central nervous system. These congenital defects are either the result of genetic influence or injurious conditions in utero. There is often great difficulty in differentiating between the two since they resemble each other closely.

The hereditary defects (genetic) are often sex linked and usually cause malformations of the pyramidal tract and cerebellum (Denhoff, 1951) and are either static or progressive in nature. In the static type of defect the anomalies are present at birth and do not increase in severity, but with the progressive type they are often not obvious at birth but manifest themselves later (as evidenced in the study of Corah *et al.* (1965)).

Prenatal anoxia

Anoxia is probably the most important potential cause of injury to which the embryo and developing foetus are exposed (Courville, 1953; Ingalls, 1950; Workany, 1950) since oxygen in an adequate supply is essential for the normal development and function of all tissues and organs. While anoxia for a short period of time might not prove injurious, the effects of a long deprivation are very serious, the brain in particular being the organ most sensitive to such deprivation.

Authorities differ as to the effect that anoxia has on brain injury. As Potter (1952) states:

> The effect of anoxia on an infant during neonatal or foetal life who subsequently survives is difficult to determine. The only changes ordinarily ascribed to anoxia are cerebral, and it is usually impossible to be certain that other changes in the Central Nervous System, such as gross haemorrhage or malformations may not have been co-existent and responsible for the major symptoms.

Before birth the baby is entirely dependent on the mother for its oxygen supply, which reaches it through the placenta and umbilical cord. If it is to survive, the foetus must have a supply which is adequate and a circulation competent enough to carry it, the cord and placenta must be reasonably normal and the baby must have no abnormality which prevents him from utilising it.

Blood vessels like other tissues require oxygen if they are to function normally, therefore if a serious lack of oxygen occurs the lining of the capillary walls may be damaged, especially in premature babies whose vessels are not as strong as full term babies. The result is that the vessels rupture and blood seeps through, the degree of haemorrhage depending on the severity of the anoxia. Whenever bleeding occurs the pressure caused leads to injury in adjacent areas, the bleeding causes further anoxia and thus a vicious circle is set up. The resulting clinical syndrome depends upon the extent of the bleeding, the part of the brain which is injured and the developmental status and general condition of the baby.

Virus infection

Because a virus is so small, it depends on the cells for its nourishment, and multiplies within the cells themselves, resulting in either malfunction or death of the cell. With this pattern of existence viruses can thus pass all around the body in the blood. Thus if infection occurs early in pregnancy, the virus may enter the blood, cross the placenta and settle in the foetus. The virus may then cause the death of the foetus or may just localise in certain tissues and damage sensitive cells causing certain defects. On the other hand, the virus may cross late and invade the tissues of the foetus, resulting in the birth of the child with the same clinical features as the mother, e.g. smallpox and chickenpox. The virus infections which could cause damage are: pneumonia, colds, polio, encephalitis, rubella, chickenpox, smallpox, mumps, measles, and influenza.

Rubella (German measles) is a particularly damaging infection if transmitted to the embryo in the first trimester. After this vital period of organ differentiation the foetus seems to be much less prone to damage. The three major abnormalities caused by rubella are congenital cataract, heart disease and deafness.

Primary prevention against rubella entails contracting the illness either by infection from another person so that antibodies are set up within the potential mother's body, or by immunisation with gamma globulin, which has a similar effect without the patient actually suffering the illness. In Australia, where the association between congenital malformation and rubella was first noticed, primary prevention is taken very seriously and as Chamberlain (1969) reports, 'Rubella camps' have been set up:

> These are holiday camps where young girls can live for two weeks away from the rest of the community but in contact with the disease. Rubella is so contagious that it spreads rapidly through all the campers; it is so mild that it rarely spoils the holidays for more than a couple of days.

If rubella is diagnosed during a pregnancy, secondary prevention is something of an 'all or nothing' matter. It is doubtful whether immunisation would be of any avail since the infection would have crossed the placenta by the time the symptoms appeared in the mother, if indeed they appeared at all. If infection has occurred in the first trimester there is a significant likelihood of damage to the embryo and thereapeutic abortion must be considered as a secondary preventative measure.

The Rhesus factor

There is some concern when a rhesus negative (Rh−) mother bears a child from a rhesus positive (Rh+) father. The likelihood is that the child will be Rh+ in which case there will be an incompatibility of blood groups, and the mother may form antibodies against the other blood group. Usually in the first pregnancy there are insufficient of these antibodies formed to harm the child. With each successive pregnancy, the numbers increase, with the result that eventually the foetal blood has too many to cope with.

Thus when the infant is born many of the blood cells are of an immature type known as erythroblasts (erythroblastosis foetalis). This may result in the child being born with, or soon developing, anaemia and usually jaundice; the jaundice may involve the brain in which case the condition is known as kernicterus.

It has been suggested by Weiner (1946) and Zeulzer (1950) that there is a positive correlation between the severity of the signs of erythroblastosis during the neonatal period, and the occurrence later of neurological sequelae. Therefore both to save infant lives and to prevent neurological after effects,

Weiner concludes that all babies with seriologically proved erythroblastosis due to Rh+ sensitisation should be treated immediately after birth with an exchange transfusion of Rh− blood.

Toxaemias of pregnancy

Toxaemia of pregnancy refers to a poisoned state of the blood which is detrimental to the health of the mother and foetus. Pre-eclampsia and eclampsia are possibly the best known.

Pre-eclampsia is characterised by the appearance in the second half of pregnancy of three signs: oedema or excessive weight gain, hypertension (increased blood pressure) and albuminuria (a condition characterised by the presence in the urine of various proteins—usually a sign of kidney trouble). The condition leads to a placental insufficiency, and this may cause an impairment of the nutritional supply of the foetus, producing amongst other things smaller babies than normal. There is a drop in the production of the sex hormones oestrogen and progesterone, but an increase in the production of the hormone gonadotrophin. There may be a swelling of the kidneys with an accompanying increase in serum uric acid, which can cause small cerebral lesions. With the swelling the efficiency of the glomerual filtration drops instead of increasing, and due to this inefficiency there is an increase in fluid and salt content.

Eclampsia is characterised by similar conditions but accompanied by a convulsion of an epileptic type.

The foetus may suffer in one or two ways, either it may die or be damaged in utero at any stage of the disease, or it may die or be damaged if induced prematurely for maternal safety reasons.

The total foetal loss is around 12% made up of 7% deaths in utero, 2% of inter-natal deaths (mainly by asphyxiation) and 3% of deaths after delivery.

Climate and foetal damage

Knobloch & Passamanick (1959b) carried out some extensive research into the effect of climate on the foetus, and found that children born in the winter months stood in greater risk of damage in utero, and for a cause they hypothesised that during the third month when development was at its height the foetus was affected by reduction in the maternal protein, heat, or by stress on the hypothalamus, pituitary and cortical systems.

They also found a higher proportion of pregnancy complications for those winter births and that the hotter the summer the more mental defectives produced.

Cigarette smoking

Smithells & Morgan (1970) report,

> The relationship between *cigarette smoking* in pregnancy and reduced birth weight is now well established and it appears reasonably certain that the weight reduction is directly attributable to the smoking and is not due to any associated factor. Even as few as five cigarettes a day will have a detectable effect on foetal growth.

Buncher (1969) suggests a significant shortening of the gestation period in the order of 30 hours in mothers who smoke '1 pack a day'. He found that shortened gestation and lighter birth weight were only weakly associated with one another, were both strongly associated with smoking, and were not strongly associated with other socioeconomic and environmental variables:

> A causal relationship might be explained by a vasoconstrictive effect of nicotine on the placental blood vessels, by a higher concentration of carbon monoxide in the blood, by a smaller placenta, by increased anoxia, and so forth.

Scott-Russell (1969) found that smoking caused a reduction in maternal blood pressure and suggested that this might mask other difficulties which usually manifest themselves with rises in blood pressure. Thus there appears to be conflicting hypotheses as to the agency through which smoking causes lowered birth weight, but Scott-Russell is convinced that smoking does retard foetal development. He found that the growth of children of smokers had not caught up with that of non-smokers after a year of life. He also suggests that the effects of smoking follow the continuum of reproductive casualty resulting in 8 in 1,000 foetal deaths on one hand, and no effect upon a sturdy foetus in the other. Put another way he thinks that (Scott-Russell, 1969):

> 2 out of every 10 unsuccessful pregnancies in women who

smoke regularly would have been successful if the mother had not been a regular smoker.

Prenatal effects

Prematurity

Prematurity is probably one of the chief predisposing factors if not a direct cause of brain injury. In various studies on children with cerebral palsy, Lilienfeld *et al.* (1953), Greenspan *et al.* (1953) and Dunsdon (1952) showed that 22%, 33% and 35% respectively were found to have been premature babies compared with a national average of 1%.

A child is considered to be premature if its birth weight is 2,500 gm. or less, and the incidence varies between 4% and 10%, depending—according to Drillien (1957)—upon the social and economic status of the mother.

He lists the three main causes as pre-eclampsic toxaemia (36%), placenta praevia (15%) and hypertension (17%).

The possible causes of damage accompanying prematurity are headed by disorders of the pulmonary aeration system accounting for about 66% of deaths (Donald, 1958).

Anaemia is a common condition in prematurity, for large doses of iron are usually laid down in the last weeks of pregnancy. Donald (1958) states:

> Jaundice follows leading to Kernicterus, and even lower levels of this in the premature infant's brain may be responsible for the lowering of intelligence and the impairment of performance.

In a survey by Knobloch (1956) it is indicated that there is an overall likelihood of neurological abnormality of 8% in premature babies as against 1·6% in mature controls, the proportion tending to be inversely proportional to the weight.

Placenta Praevia

Normally a placenta is situated in the upper segment of the uterus, but with the condition placenta praevia it is situated in various positions in the lower segment; this might be due to the ovum being embedded and developing lower down in the uterine cavity.

It seems that little is known of the aetiology of the low implantation of the placenta, but it occurs more often in multi-rather than primagravidae with an incidence of roughly 1 in 80.

There is a continuum from partial to complete placenta praevia in which the placenta passes right over the internal os, to cover a large area of the lower segment all around the opening of the cervix. With this condition there is likely to be rupture of the placenta and haemorrhage constituting a real danger both to mother and foetus.

The main causes of injury to the foetus are inter-uterine asphyxia due to placental separation and hypertension in the mother. The hazards of delivery are increased for there is often mal-presentation of the infant who is any way more prone to inter-cranial haemorrhage.

Precipitate labour

Unusually rapid labour may be due to either too frequent or to powerful contractions of the uterus, or to a lower uterine segment that dilates with unusual ease. The vigorous contractions are not necessarily associated with pain and so the patient may be in labour for some time without realising it.

The dangers of precipitate labour are the obvious injury to the foetus or rupture of the umbilical cord if the mother is not prone when delivered. The rapid expulsion of the head may result in tentorial tearing with intercranial haemorrhage and frequent violent uterine contractions. With only short intervals of relaxation this may lead to degrees of asphyxia.

Pelvic deformity

Deformities in the pelvis can be considered as those due to disease, congenital defects or abnormalities of the spine.

Ricketts often leads to a flattening of the pelvic opening, whilst other causative factors are polio, tuberculosis, arthritis of the hip and congenital dislocation of the hip. Abnormalities of the spine such as scoliosis often lead to assymmetry of the pelvis.

Anomalies in presentation

Breech presentations

A breech presentation is favoured by anything which prevents the head from engaging in the pelvic outlet: contracted pelvis, placenta praevia, an excess of liquor amnii, hydroencephally, prematurity or twin pregnancy.

D

If the usual attitude of flexion of the lower limbs is maintained presenting part consists of buttocks and feet, the position being described as a fully flexed breech and is the commonest in multigravidae.

If while the thighs remain flexed on the trunk, the legs are extended at the knee joint, the presenting part consists of buttocks only, a position most common in primagravidae and termed Extended Legs or Frank Breech.

If the legs remain flexed but the thighs extend, the knees present and if both legs and thighs extend then the feet present, both of the latter presentations being rare.

There are many other anomalies of presentation concerning the upper half of the body. Occasionally a shoulder will present, with various degrees of mal-presentation, the head sometimes appears facing the wrong way and this is termed a Brow Presentation.

The normal course of pregnancy sees the foetus turning a somersault at about the 34th week of development. The anomalies arise when this movement is prevented or impeded.

It is more dangerous for the baby to be born breech first than by the normal vertex position for it may die from asphyxia, due to the head being delivered too slowly. Directly the head enters the pelvic brim the cord is obstructed between the head and the brim, whilst the baby cannot breath itself until the mouth and nose are delivered.

By far the most common injury and cause of death is due to inter-cranial haemorrhage caused by the head being delivered too quickly. In the normal vertex delivery the head takes hours to pass through the bony pelvis and has plenty of time to accommodate itself to the rigid canal. Moreover passing through the pelvic floor and the vulva the pressures all the time tend to draw the cranial vault away from the base of the skull. This in turn leads to a tear in the tentorium and is the primary cause of haemorrhage.

Forceps deliveries

Forceps are used in deliveries where there is delay in the second stage of labour (which is the passage of the baby's head through the birth canal and into the world), foetal asphyxia and any adverse maternal indications.

Delay is most often due to inefficient contractions of the

uterus, abnormal resistance of the pelvic floor or to mal-presentation of the occiput.

Maternal indications are often the sole reason for forceps and it is thought better to deliver the foetus than to let the mother become exhausted in the second stage of labour. In normal women an indication to deliver by forceps is if the head's progress ceases or if delivery has not occurred two hours after complete dilation of the cervix. In special cases it is thought that an easy forceps delivery does less harm than a prolonged second stage.

The technique of applying the forceps to the head of the foetus and inducing traction is extremely critical, for increase in pressure on the skull and extension of the spinal cord during rotation can have serious repercussions such as inter-cranial haemorrhage, tentorial tearing of the pia-arachnoid tissue. There is also the ever present danger in high forceps deliveries, that the forceps will trap the cord thus denuding the foetus of the placental blood supply.

There is also the danger that in manipulating the presenting limbs, to facilitate an easier birth the nerve plexus might be damaged, resulting in loss or impairment of limb control.

Caesarian section

A caesarian section consists of removal of the foetus from the uterus by an incision through the wall of the uterus and is performed either in the upper (Classical) or lower segment.

It is normally performed if certain indications are present: extreme disproportion; e.g. if gross pelvic contraction exists, antepartum haemorrhage, with placenta praevia if the conditions are suitable. Often malpresentation can be dealt with in some other way but in the case of a shoulder, brow or face presentation caesarian is nearly always the choice if other simple procedures are ineffective.

Other conditions leading to a section are: extreme delay in dilation of the cervix, uterine inertia, prolapse of the cord, foetal anoxia and serious illness of the mother.

The risks to the baby are from the operation itself, and are largely those of anaesthesia and asphyxia due to the administration of anaesthetics to the mother and the resultant maternal asphyxia being passed to the foetus.

The damage risk is increased in prematurity, since often the operation is performed before term, when the organs and tissues are not fully developed, thus rapid pressure changes can lead to haemorrhages, the lungs not being fully developed, respiratory difficulties become evident.

Twin pregnancies

Twin pregnancies are said to be a factor in predisposing brain injury, and the second born child is thought to be more likely to be affected. The first part of the statement seems to be unquestioned, but the latter has not been confirmed in more recent studies. Potter (1952) found that the mortality rate for the first and second born twins, if one excludes the long dead macerated foetus, which are usually second born, were equal.

Among a hundred cases selected at random at Lennox Hill C.P. Clinic, Greenspan & Deaver (1953) found six representatives of pairs of twins, compared with a general incidence of one pair of twins in every eighty-five deliveries. Most twin pregnancies are premature, so prematurity rather than twin pregnancies might be the important causative factor in the high mortality.

Complications of pregnancy particularly pre-eclampsia, post-partum haemorrhage or an excess of liquor amnii are more frequently found in twin than in single pregnancies. Malformations incompatible with life were found to be slightly higher in twin than in single pregnancies.

The possible effects of pre- and paranatal damage on motor ability

Brain disorders as they affect motor performance directly represent a syndrome known as cerebral palsy. As Perlstein (1952) states:

> Cerebral Palsy is a term used to designate any paralysis, weakness or inco-ordination, or functional abberation of the motor system resulting from brain injury. Lesions in different parts of the brain produce different symptoms of motor dysfunction. Five common types have been identified: Spastic, Athetoid, Rigidity, Ataxic, Tremor. In addition many subtypes especially of the Athetoids have been described.

It is well at this stage to indicate that the disorders to be described are the gross cases. The cases that most educationalists are likely to come across are obviously the mild forms of such conditions.

The classification of cerebral palsy has two main forms, that of the condition and that of the topography of the disorder.

Spasticity

The neuromuscular condition that characterises spasticity is an increase in the stretch reflex. In addition there is an increase in the muscle tone of the spastic muscles and a weakness in those muscles in opposition to it.

It is usually possible for the individual to move the affected muscle voluntarily, but the motion may be explosive, jerky, slow or poorly performed. The muscle itself is normal unless the prolonged contraction against weak or flaccid opposing muscles has caused permanent contracture (Perlstein, 1961).

Because of the hyper-active stretch reflexes and slow contraction time the movements of the spastic are poorly coordinated. The tendency for the anti-gravity muscles to maintain a state of contraction, and for the antagonists to lengthen correspondingly, produces characteristic flexion deformities, particularly at the large joints. There is a small group of children called atonic spastics whose characteristic is muscular weakness rather than spasticity.

It appears that this exaggerated stretch reflex is associated with upper motor-neuron lesions.

Chorea

This is an acute toxic disorder of the nervous system usually due to acute rheumatism, occurring in childhood and adolescence, being characterised by involuntary movements.

Apart from rheumatism the causes could be scarlet fever and diphtheria, whilst choreiform movements may be a symptom of encaphalitis or a complication of chickenpox.

Heredity may play some part in the aetiology since some families appear to be unusually susceptible to rheumatism and there may be a family history of either chorea or rheumatic manifestation.

Over-work at school may be a predisposing factor and it is not uncommon for the onset of an attack to be associated with fright.

The involuntary movements are of a high order and semi-purposive with eyes rolling and bizarre movements of the tongue and mouth.

In the upper limbs movements occur at all joints. Respiration is often jerky and frequently impeded, with movements accentuated by effort or excitement which disappear with sleep and thus have no deforming effect.

Ataxia

The Ataxic's muscles are normal although there may at times be some weakness. There is no spasticity or involuntary motions and reflexes are normal. The distinguishing characteristic of the Ataxic is the disturbance of equilibrium. His righting reflex is diminished and his sense of position in space is disturbed. Often the condition is not noticed until the child begins to walk.

It is thought that as the cerebellum is involved in various phases of synergic muscle action and cereballar lesions affect the regularity of muscle action, then it is the damage to the cerebellum that causes Ataxia.

Tremor

The muscles of the tremor type of cerebral palsy are normal in tone and there are no abnormal reflexes. The distinguishing neuromuscular characteristic is repetitive rhythmic involuntary contractions of flexor and extensor muscles. The tremors may be intentional or unintentional and differ from the athetoid in being fine and rhythmic. Tremors in the lower extremities may throw the person off balance, whilst tremors in the upper extremities interfere with hand skills, often with fine movements such as writing. The tremor type does not develop any deformity and again the cerebellum is thought to be responsible.

Rigidity

The distinguishing neuromuscular characteristic of rigidity is resistance to flexion and extension movements, resulting from simultaneous contraction of both the agonist and antagonist muscle groups. Attempts to move a limb are often described as like trying to bend a lead pipe. The rigidity can be constant or intermittent, the former leading to deformities. Because of the simultaneous contraction of both agonists and antagonists, the person is only capable of slow movements within a restricted range (Deaver, 1952).

Mixed

Some of the conditions described singly occur in the presence of others. Spastics for example may be found to have some weak, non-spastic muscles or even normal muscles.

Classification according to topography

Cerebral palsy may also be defined according to the location and number of limbs involved. The three most common classifications are hemiplegia, paraplegia and quadraplegia.

In paraplegia the legs only are involved, and the condition is rarely found in any but spastic cases.

In quadraplegia or tetraplegia both arms and both legs are involved, but involvement of the legs is more severe in spastics although the quadraplegia might be an athetoid tremor or rigidity type.

In triplegia the extremities, both the legs and one arm are involved. Such cases are usually spastic, and may be combinations of hemiplegia and paraplegia.

Brain dysfunction

Because of the generality and diverse possibilities covered by this term it can best be elaborated by cross references from a number of studies. Clarke (1966) has made a useful start by analogy with a TV set. He suggests that the best evidence of dysfunction in such a set is an examination of the picture it produces, i.e. the output of the whole machine. If the machine is deficient, it is possible to dismantle the set and test the integrity of each physical component. They may all be found to be sound, i.e. the fault may be due to a deficit in assembly. Clarke's point is that negative findings from such investigations cannot exclude brain dysfunction.

Stott (1966) in formulating what is perhaps the latest developed test of motor impairment rejects the term 'minimal' brain damage as being too all-embracing in its references as to the cause of motor impairment and prefers to substitute the term 'neural dysfunction' as this term is less exclusive of other possible causal factors.

Gubbay et al. (1965) are clearly against classifying all instances of impairment as being the result of brain damage. While in their study of clumsy children, the E.E.G. examination together with high incidence of perinatal abnormality suggested underlying brain damage in many cases, in others, they suggest a fundamentally disordered physiology. They conclude that various types of apraxia and agnosia are of congenital origin or arise in infancy and may be quite unassociated with any other collateral clinical evidence of brain damage.

Walton *et al.* (1962) explain that in some cases the clinical picture would appear to reflect a cerebral disorganisation in a neurophysiological rather than an anatomical sense. A developmental deficit was suggested by Ford (1959) to account for what he terms 'congenital maladroitness' in intelligent children who are slow to learn complex motor skills. Drew (1956) in a study of three cases of familial dyslexia concluded that although all three subjects displayed different combinations of defects in directional selection, mixed hand-eye dominance, face-hand test abnormalities and spatial disorientation they could all be viewed as showing variant manifestations of a fundamental defect in correct 'figure-ground' recognition due to some fault in parietal lobe development.

Fish (1961) is even more explicit in reporting on a study concerned with eighty-five 12-year-old impaired children whom she had been treating over a period of 7 years.

She suggests that:

> Immaturity and poor organisation of functions under the control of the C.N.S. can be seen in tests of motility, perception, intelligence and in the E.E.G. Disorders of these functions are found in children with known brain damage and in a large number of children whose behaviour disorders are accompanied by less specific impairments but who resemble brain-damaged children in their hyperactivity, impulsivity, and low threshold for anxiety.

The concept of brain dysfunction will be returned to in considering sensory, perceptual and movement deprivation as this would appear to involve learning difficulties.

It would be difficult to be explicit as to the reasons for brain dysfunction. It is a developmental deficit which can be multideterminined. Reference once again to the system model in Chapter 1 gives some idea of the complexity of the systems which need to be developed for effective performance and the way in which they interrelate but even this is painting a very much oversimplified picture. Beer (1960) questions the whole 'black-box' approach to the organisation of behaviour and while not sharing completely his scepticism, his comments are both relevant and salutary:

There are rectangles representing activities, or processes or operations, or even people. In information theory terms, the amount of variety denoted by each box may be colossal. The boxes are solemnly connected by attenuated, solitary lines with arrowheads on the ends. (What channel capacity those lines must have!) Now, three questions: How many vital features of the organic wholeness of the system have been utterly obliterated by this particular division? How many essential relationships between each bit in each box are depicted by the connections shown, and (given that this is a well understood convention) have we any means of recognising the condition in which one of those not shown will turn this version of the system into another and quite different version? Can the passage of information (in however a subtle interpretation) really account for the wholeness of the whole, or is there something yet to learn from Hegel about other models of relatedness?

It has already been suggested that some children will be born with inherently less potential for development such that when compared with children of a similar age they will always appear retarded. In addition, children born with the normal potential must encounter an environment suitable for the development of such potential. In many ways this means simply the provision of an environment where the maximum possible opportunity for sensory, perceptual and movement experience is available since it would be difficult to know exactly what environment to fit to each child. To a large extent, knowledge in this area is based on negative findings from the many studies carried out on sensory, perceptual and movement deprivation. Unfortunately, it is often necessary to refer to animal studies since those for human beings are limited in the main to observation of the effects of particularly unfavourable environments it being difficult and undesirable to structure experimental studies in which one group of children is systematically deprived of experience. While results from animal studies may not be directly relevant, it is interesting that Bronfenbrenner (1968) after carrying out a cross species analysis of early deprivation declared himself to be surprised at the amount of generality to be found. He suggested that the most surprising and possibly sobering outcome of his detailed comparative analysis was the similarity humans bear to their fellow primates, at least when it comes to the need for stimulation and for attachment to others. The effects of early experience have proved to be of significance in monkey, dog, cat, guinea pig, rat and mouse as well as in fish and fowl.

Hebb (1949) in particular has propounded a theory which predicts that animals that have had a large amount of perceptual experience early in life will prove better learners than others deprived of such experience. The magnitude of such a facilitative effect is within rough limits inversely related to the age at which the perceptual experience is gained (Beach & Jaynes, 1954).

Although evidence from the field of human behaviour is less conclusive than that from the animal world, it has only recently been appreciated how important for mental development are the effects of early experience. Hebb (1966) proposes that sensory stimulation from the early environment is necessary for the maintenance of some neural structures which would otherwise degenerate and also for the occurrence of learning which is essential for normal adult behaviour. Early experience is said to build up the 'mediating processes' (neural activity of the brain which can hold the excitation delivered by a sensory event after this event has ceased) which once established make possible the very rapid learning of the mature adult. Hebb (1949) suggests the formation of cell-assemblies—hypothetical reverberating systems within the brain—as the basis of such mediating processes.

Postnatal effects

Sensory, Perceptual and Movement Deprivation

It is clear from the examination of evidence from some of the more extreme studies, that gross deprivation of one kind or another can result in impaired performance which at some later stage will give rise to levels of performance which are maladaptive. This applies not only to those skills in which learning plays a major role but also to those skills which have perhaps inaptly been termed 'maturational skills'. The idea of maturational skills in which learning plays a limited part and is only appropriate when a particular level of maturation has been reached is an accepted category of skilled behaviour. Of particular interest in this respect are the locomotive skills on which so much later gross body skill learning depends. It is not possible on the basis of current information to assess the limitations of retardation in the development of such skills on later skill learning or on development in general or whether such limitations are transitory in nature. The classical study illustrating the limitation of practice on children learning to walk, is Dennis's (1940) description of the Hopi Indians who bind their children on to cradle-boards for most of the day. These children apparently develop the ability to sit, creep and walk just as rapidly as children who are never bound. What is often missed in such explanations is the opportunity for other learning and development which is possible under such restrictions. It would appear for example that one of the reasons for binding children on to cradle-boards is that they can be carried on the mother's back. It is to be assumed therefore that such children do not suffer the perceptual (at least visual, auditory and haptic) deprivation which is the lot of children in more restricted environments. The point being made here, is that the concept of maturation applies to the organism *as a whole* and is not specific to some part of it.

Schaffer & Emerson (1968) make the further suggestion that:

> . . . the sheer weight of evidence has been such as to give strong support to the view that early development is not just a maturational unfolding of inherent capacities at predetermined rates, but is based on processes occurring in the context of environmental conditions that may foster or impede the individual's progress to varying degrees.

Because it is the norm for children to walk at particular ages for example in a given culture, it should not be assumed that particularly favourable opportunities to learn in the general sense might not accelerate the potential age at which walking is possible or particularly unfavourable conditions put back the age. The same reasoning could be applied to other 'maturational' skills. This point is well made by comparing the Geber (1958) studies on native reared Baganda children who show precocious motor behaviour (including walking) in the first eighteen months of life and some of Spitz's (1958) findings on institutionalised children. According to Geber, the Baganda children walk *on average* at ten months of age. Spitz on the other hand followed up twenty-one children who remained in a foundling home up to four years of age. Of these, the youngest was two and the oldest four years and one month. Only five of the twenty-one could walk unassisted, eight could walk with assistance, three could sit-up but not walk and five were incapable of locomotion. These children had suffered severe sensory and perceptual deprivation which presumably had delayed the maturational process.

Variations in the onset of a maturational phase conducive to walking which would be difficult to interpret in terms of genetic endowment can be found if an attempt is made to quote European norms for the onset of walking behaviour which can be contrasted with those of the native-reared Baganda. Significant discrepancies were found by Hindley et al. (1966) in a longitudinal study of age of first walking in five European samples (Table 1). There were no significant sex or social class differences within any of the samples. Presumably, therefore, the observed differences represent underlying population variations which might be genetic, environmental or combinations of the two. This reinforces the difficulty previously described of universal standards for both motor performance and impairment.

The literature on deprivation is vast and it would be pointless attempting to survey what has been done so much more thoroughly in texts such as Newton & Levine (1968). Some of the issues in this respect have been raised and what follows represents a selection of viewpoints and evidence considered to be particularly applicable to the problem of motor impairment.

One of the difficulties of putting a more specific interpretation on laboratory experimental studies, is that of isolating the contribution of the factors of sensory, perceptual and movement experience. In restricting the opportunity for perceptual experience, it is generally necessary to restrict opportunities for movement—particularly if proprioception is linked with perception.* Again, it is difficult to restrict movement alone without also restricting perceptual experience. Two experiments in particular employed experimental designs which attempted the difficult task of independent assessment of the role of movement and these will serve to illustrate the point.

*Bernhaut et al. (1953) for example maintain that kinesthetic stimuli are even more important that visual or auditory stimuli for reticular excitation. (An activation/arousal concept of this nature was raised in the last chapter and will be returned to later.)

Kulka et al. (1960) have proposed that rocking and head banging and other such rhythmic movements which are seen in infants with prolonged deprivation may be an attempt to gratify their own kinesthetic needs.

TABLE 1

Age of walking by sex and social class in each sample (Hindley et al. (1966))
All values are in terms of logarithm of age in months except the last two
columns, which are in months (S.D.'s × 100)

	Social class	Boys			Girls			Total sample			
		N	Mean	S.D. (×100)	N	Mean	S.D. (×100)	Mean	S.D. (×100)	Mean (months)	Median (months)
Brussels N = 211	1 & 2	42	1·118	6·99	34	1·108	6·46	1·102	6·34	12·65	12·48
	3	48	1·109	6·75	42	1·089	5·49				
	4 & 5	25	1·089	5·50	20	1·095	5·76				
London N = 152	1 & 2	12	1·162	6·16	10	1·128	12·57	1·124	7·40	13·31	13·23
	3	24	1·111	6·59	21	1·106	6·27				
	4 & 5	39	1·121	6·51	46	1·131	7·78				
Paris N = 272	1 & 2	18	1·132	4·39	20	1·146	6·92	1·140	7·33	13·81	13·58
	3	58	1·144	6·13	43	1·138	6·92				
	4 & 5	71	1·138	8·01	62	1·141	8·63				
Stockholm N = 209	1 & 2	29	1·104	5·01	21	1·100	5·92	1·097	6·45	12·51	12·44
	3	39	1·099	6·97	26	1·095	6·38				
	4 & 5	52	1·096	7·02	42	1·093	6·70				
Zurich N = 233	1 & 2	32	1·122	6·65	25	1·142	5·06	1·134	5·65	13·59	13·63
	3	81	1·136	5·54	78	1·132	5·52				
	4 & 5	5	1·125	4·90	12	1·150	6·10				

Reprinted from Human Biology, 38.4, December 1966, by C. B. Hindley, 'Age of Walking', by permission of the Wayne State University Press.

In a study of rats reared in small cages restricting body movement but not perception Hymovitch (1952) showed that such animals performed much better in maze learning than comparable animals who had been reared in enclosed activity wheels. Indeed, if the cages were moved from time to time the rats did as well in perceptual motor tests as free ones. However, Hymovitch used cages which permitted *some* movement. Forgays & Forgays (1952) found their free movement group much superior to rats raised in mesh cages which severely limited movement experience. This, taken with the importance of distance cues for maze learning suggested by Hymovitch and supported experimentally by Forgays, points to the conclusion that movement in space plays a real contribution to the development of visual function.

Although it is difficult to separate out the respective contributions of movement and perceptual deprivation, the fact that in the Hymovitch study rats restricted in cages, but whose cages were moved about, were indistinguishable from animals who had been free to move about in the environment leads to the suggestion that it is not movement restriction *per se* but the fact that the animals are being deprived of opportunity for varied perceptual experience. One further difficulty here is that the effects of movement restriction have been related to later perceptual functioning but they have not been related to later movement behaviour of a quantitative or qualitative nature.

Returning to the 'activation' hypothesis raised earlier but not previously related to the deprivation concept, Schaffer (1965) reports an interesting comparison between two groups of infants undergoing a temporary period (2–9 months) of institutionalisation. The staff-child ratio (an index of deprivation) in the 'hospitalised' group (the more deprived) was 1 : 6 and in the 'baby-home' group (an institution for children who had been in contact with T.B. though they themselves were not ill) 1 : 2·5. The hospitalised infants received minimal environmental changes in that they remained in their cots for the majority of their stay while the baby-home infants were taken from their dormitory to the gardens (where they spent some time) twice a day. The developmental quotients of the hospitalised infants were found to be significantly lower than those of the less-deprived infants. While no progressive deterioration of scores took place during institutionalisation the developmental quotients of the deprived groups jumped to the level of the other group shortly following their return home while those of the non-deprived group remained relatively constant. Schaffer interprets this temporary decrement in performance (and also in vocalisation and activity) in terms of a depressant effect on arousal due to insufficient stimulation. While maturation continues to take place (hence no progressive deterioration occurred) the failure of the environment to arouse potentially available responses results in the infant functioning below his optimal level.

In a further study, Schaffer (1966) draws attention to constitutionally determined differences in activity level and their interactions with the environment in a deprivation situation. Taking infants on a continuum of active–inactive (in terms of amount of spontaneous behaviour displayed) he was able to show that inactive infants are more likely to be adversely affected than are active infants in such situations. He maintains that the proprioceptive feedback available to the active infant will heighten its level of alertness; that such activity will lead to frequent changes in position resulting in access to new environmental stimuli and that the proprioceptive stimulation so obtained increases the responsiveness of cortical areas to afferent stimulation resulting in increased responsiveness to external sources of stimulation.

A follow-up study (Schaffer & Emerson, 1968) examined the effects of experimentally administered stimulation on the developmental quotients of infants. Results indicated that changes in developmental assessment scores can be readily produced by manipulating the amount of stimulus input to which an infant is currently exposed. Such changes are interpreted in terms of changes in arousal level. As these workers point out, young infants have only limited ability to produce self-stimulation and hence are dependent on their current environment for the necessary means to maintain arousal. They make the additional salient point that the ability of the infant to produce certain responses is dependent not only on their behavioural repertoire but on the opportunity to make such potential behaviour manifest by the maintenance of an optimal arousal level.

In view of these findings and the considerable evidence which is amassing from experimental work on sensory and perceptual deprivation, the notion of the human organism as a passive responder to stimuli is hardly tenable. The organism must be conceived as an active, aggressive seeker of stimulation (Schulz, 1965) whose development is affected in a deleterious way when deprived of opportunities to obtain such stimulation. The difference is related to Gibson's (1968) concept of *imposed perception* which occurs when the organs are passive and stimulation impinges on them and *obtained perception* which occurs when the senses are considered as perceptual systems which actively seek information.

The importance of selecting the right information from the environment as a factor in skill performance was outlined in Chapter 2. For some skills, such information will be of primary importance while in others its purpose may be simply that of indicating to the person performing the skill where it is to be carried out, its use in the actual control of the movement being minimal. While some features of such attention mechanisms would appear to be innately given and to function under the appropriate environmental conditions (Fantz, 1961), the major contribution towards the development of such systems must relate to postnatal experience. The question which must be asked, is the way in which previous experience influences selective attention and what effects deprivation in all its forms is likely to have on the development of such mechanisms. Evidence from a growing number of experimental procedures leads to the suggestion that central nervous system processes subserving memories, attention, emotional states, etc., can block, facilitate or otherwise modify sensory input patterns by means of systems of fibres that run from the brain to synaptic regions in the afferent pathways (Melzack, 1968). The most reasonable interpretation in Melzack's (1968) view is conceived as a two-part process in which (*a*) there is inadequate filtering of inputs on the basis of memories of the significance of such stimuli normally acquired in early experience so that (*b*) the total input bombarding the C.N.S. produces an excessive arousal which as Hebb (1955) has suggested could be responsible for the correspondingly low cue properties necessary for discrimination and adaptive response.

The effect of excessive deprivation of sensory, perceptual and movement experience would seem to be the lack of 'knowledge' which the person has about the significance of particular stimuli in new skill learning situations and hence the lack of a basis for selective attention to one stimulus complex rather than another. Melzack (1968) suggests that the evidence points to a failure to filter out irrelevant information on the basis of prior experience leading to excessive arousal which in turn interferes with mechanisms both innate and acquired that would normally act in the selection of cues for adaptive responses.

This brief survey of the field is sufficient for the reader to be able to understand the possible influences that sensory, perceptual and movement deprivation are likely to have not only in terms of motor impairment, but in intellectual and social development as well. It is likely that in such cases there exists a general low level of potential for learning skills in all these areas. Hebb (1966) perhaps sums the overall viewpoint appropriately when he suggests that normal development depends on a normal perceptual environment. The animal reared in isolation is a permanent screwball at maturity, motivationally, socially, intellectually abnormal.

In an attempt to differentiate between motor impairment which was the result of brain damage and that which could principally be attributed to deprivation of one form or another, Whiting et al. (1969a, 1969b) carried out two studies. The first study looked at the incidence of motor impairment in a sample of 50 E.S.N. children. The Stott (1966) test of motor impairment was used as the criterion but also in the test battery were tests purporting to assess brain damage. A high incidence of similarity was found between those children who scored very low on the Stott test and those who failed the tests of brain damage suggesting that in this population the motor impairment together with the intellectual impairment might be attributed to the effects of brain damage. In a further study on a criterion group of sixty boys from a junior approved school (Whiting et al., 1970) similar procedures were utilised. In this sample the number of children failing the Stott test on the criterion adopted was 26% but of these, very few children indeed failed on the tests of brain damage. This together with parental interviews and screening of record cards led to the suggestion that in this population brain damage would not appear to be the primary cause of impairment. It was suggested that the cause was more likely to be attributed to environmental

E

conditions involving deprivation of one kind or another. The evidence further suggested that it would be almost impossible to attribute the impairment to any one cause. A more likely interpretation was that such impairment was multi-determined with brain damage apparently affecting only a small percentage of the children.

Emotional Disturbance

The idea that psychological factors or events producing emotional stress in the mother can harm the unborn child still meets with some resistance. Yet the marked changes in the incidence of certain types of human malformation in wartime and during other times of stress seems to offer support.

A number of studies in Germany showed a marked increase in malformations during the postwar years.

During the prewar years the mean was 1·43/1,000 births, it doubled the year Hitler came to power. During the war years it was 2·6 and reached 6·5 for the years 1946–50. Employment and nutrition were better during the prewar and early war years, which leads to the theory that the mental stresses from persecution, violence and later, bombing, were responsible (Eichmann & Gesenius, 1952).

In Britain an indication of a similar trend can be seen from the statistics on the incidence per 1,000 births of infant deaths within one month of birth, the cause of which was given as malformation. The peak for both male and female deaths was during the period 1940–2 when emotional stress was great. During this time with rationing and full employment the dietary standard was probably higher than in prewar years.

In one study Stott (1962) examined the incidence of mongol births related to emotional shock, his criterion being whether or not the event experienced by the mother would have been likely to produce severe emotional upset in women of normal temperament.

He found that the incidence of accidents was spread throughout the term and thus the mongol type delivery could not be due to injury alone. This led him to believe that the shock or stress caused a hormone disturbance which led in turn to certain deficiencies.

Strengthening the argument that stress and emotional shock could affect the development of the foetus Klebanov (1948) found that the incidence of mongol births was eight times greater than normal in Jewish women just released from prison camps.

Stott concludes:

> The whole aetiology is complicated by the fact that only a very few abnormal embryos develop to foetal maturity, and by the ignorance of the process of weeding out. Hertig (1953) found that of 36 embryos examined upon hysterectomy, 36% were abnormal compared with an observed malformation rate of 1%. The process by which these nonviable foetuses are expelled or re-absorbed is probably a hormonal one. It is noteworthy that Woolan & Miller (1960) succeeded in reducing the incidence of hare lip in a strain of rats, who produce such spontaneously, by administering thyroxine. Since the effect on the latter was also to significantly reduce the fertility rate it may also have been that this hormone aids in the weeding out of imperfect embryos. It may be speculatively suggested as an additional possible alternative that severe emotional shock, by disturbing endocrine balance, interferes with the mechanism possibly hormonal, through which the weeding out is implemented; in other words, but for these shocks the mongol children would never have been born.

Social class

The higher incidence of impairment of all kinds amongst children whose parents are classified in the lower social classes has long been appreciated. The position is particularly well illustrated in a report by Fairweather & Illsley (1960) on all the mentally handicapped children born in Aberdeen in 1948 and still living there in 1958. The fifty-eight mothers concerned were interviewed, the interview ranging over the social, educational occupational background of the parents and siblings of the child, the mother's obstetric history and the child's own education and health, particular attention being paid to illnesses and accidents which might have affected the child's mental development.

The pregnancy and labour records showed that in eight cases, complications had arisen (one forceps delivery responsible for cerebral damage, three cases of hazard from placental insufficiency which may have caused brain damage, and four cases of obstetric abnormality (no details)). Of the cases, twelve had been born weighing $5\frac{1}{2}$ lb. or less and the prematurity rate was 16·9%. This is very high compared with the norm for Aberdeen which is 5·6%. There was a strong tendency for these women who produced one premature child to bear small babies in other pregnancies. The premature mentally handicapped children had 31 siblings of whom 10 (32%) were also premature; the full weight children had 183 siblings of whom only 9 (5%) were premature. In general then, the mentally handicapped series contained an excess of children who were premature by weight at birth and of mothers who gave birth to more than one premature child. The social history of the families of the premature children showed a close association between obstetric and social factors.

Mental handicap as already suggested, is closely associated with physical defects, some congenital, some arising through childhood illness and some of indeterminate origin. In twenty-one of the children a specific physical defect was identified— two mongols, one cerebral palsy due to birth injury, four cases of epilepsy, one case of microcephaly, two had severe impediments of speech, one had two years in hospital with osteochondritis. In the ten remaining cases the link between illness and mental handicap is conjectural, although four had been in hospital as babies with febrile convulsions and in two growth was severely retarded. The ten children with the lowest IQ all appeared among the twenty-one children with physical handicaps or a possible predisposing illness.

An examination of the social factors involved showed that with only one exception, the mentally handicapped children came from the poorest and least stable section of the population. The mothers also came from very large families themselves (41% in families of seven or more children). Five children were illegitimate and in nine other cases the mother had borne at least one other illegitimate child. One quarter of the mothers had had a child before the age of 20 and in 1958 the mean family size was 4·7 compared with 3·3 in the rest of Scotland. So far, the 58 mothers have produced 241 siblings of whom 183 have married and produced 582 children leaving the original 58 with 843 grandchildren.

Irrespective of obstetric injury, the data suggest that low IQ has genetic origins. Numerically, prematurity appeared to be the greatest source of mental handicap.

References

Beach, F. A. & Jaynes, J. (1954) Effects of early experience upon the behaviour of animals. *Psychol. Bull.*, 51, 3, 239–263.

Bernhaut, M., Gellhorn, E. & Rasmussen, A. T. (1953) Experimental contributions to problems of consciousness. *J. Neurophysiol.*, 16, 21–35.

Beer, S. (1960) Below the twilight arch—a mythology of systems. In L. Von Bertalanffy & A. Rapoport (Eds.) *General Systems*, 5, 9–20.

Buncher, C. R. (1969) Cigarette smoking and duration of pregnancy. *Am. J. Obstet. Gynec.*, 103, 942–946.

Bronfenbrenner, U. (1968) Early deprivation in mammals. In G. Newton & S. Levine (Eds.) *Early experience and behaviour.* Springfield: Thomas.

Caldwell, V. (1956) *Advances in understanding cerebral palsy.* New York: New River Press.

Chamberlain, G. (1969) *The safety of the unborn child.* Harmondsworth: Penguin.

Clarke, P. R. F. (1966) *The nature and consequences of brain lesions in children and adults.* Proceedings of a course held by the English Division of professional psychologists. London: British Psych. Soc.

Corah, N. L., Anthony, E. J., Painter, P., Stern, J. A. & Thurston, D. L. (1965) Effects of perinatal anoxia after seven years. *Psych. Monog.*, 79, 3, 1–33.

Courville, C. B. (1953) *Contributions to the study of cerebral palsy.* Los Angeles: San Lucas Press.

Deaver, G. (1952) Etiologic factors in cerebral palsy. *Bull. New York Acad. Med.*, 28, 37–52.

Denhoff, E. (1951) Medical progress—cerebral palsy. *New England J. Med.*, 245, 728–735.

Dennis, W. (1940) The effect of cradling practices upon the onset of walking in Hopi children. *J. of Genet. Psych.*, 56, 77–86.

Donague, G. T. & Nichtern, S. (1965) *Teaching the troubled child.* New York: Free Press.

Drillien, C. N. (1957) *Jr. Obst. Gyn. Brit. Emp.*, 64, 161.

Donald, I. (1958) *Scottish Med. J.*, 3, 151.

Dunsdon, M. I. (1952) *The educability of the brain injured child.* London: National Foundation for Educational Research.

Eichmann, R. & Gesenius, W. (1952) *Arch. Gynac.*, 181, 186.

Fairweather, O. V. & Illsley, R. (1960) Obstetric and social origins of mentally handicapped children. *Brit. J. Prev. Soc. Med.*, 14, 149–159.

Fantz, R. L. (1961)   The origin of form perception. In S. Cooper-smith (Ed.) *Frontiers of psychological research*. London: Freeman.

Fish, B. (1961)   The study of motor development in infancy and its relation to psychological functioning. *Am. J. Psychiat.*, 17, 1, 113–118.

Ford, F. R. (1959)   *Diseases of the nervous system in infancy, childhood and adolescence*. Springfield: Thomas.

Forgays, O. G. & Forgays, J. W. (1952)   The nature of the effect of free environmental experience in the rat. *J. Comp. Physiol. Psych.*, 45, 322–328.

Geber, M. (1958)   The psychomotor development of African children in the first year and the influence of maternal behaviour. *J. Soc. Psych.*, 47, 185–195.

Gibson, J. J. (1968)   *The senses considered as perceptual systems*. London: George Allen & Unwin.

Greenspan, H. Leon, R. & Deaver, G. (1953)   Clinical approach to the aetiology of cerebral palsy. *Arch. Phys. Med. Rehab.*, 34, 478–485.

Gubbay, S. S., Ellis, E., Walton, J. N. & Court, S. D. M. (1965)   A study of apraxic and agnosic defects in 21 children. *J. of Neur.*, 88.

Hebb, D. O. (1949)   Organisation of behaviour. New York: Wiley.

Hebb, D. O. (1955)   Drives and the C.N.S. *Psych. Rev.*, 62, 243–254.

Hebb, D. O. (1966)   *A textbook of psychology*. Philadelphia: Saunders.

Hertig, A. T. (1953)   Traumatic abortion and prenatal death of the embryo. Report of Conference for aid of crippled children, New York.

Heyns, O. S. (1963)   *Abdominal decompression*. Johannesburg: Witwatersrand Univ. Press.

Hill, D. U., Galloway & Hughes (1958)   Virus diseases in pregnancy and congenital defects. *Brit. J. Prev. Soc. Med.*, 12, 1–7.

Hindley, C. B., Filliozat, A. M., Klackenberg, G., Nicolet-Meisten, D. & Sand, E. A. (1966)   Differences in age of walking in five European longitudinal samples. *Human Biology*, 38, 4.

Hymovitch, B. (1952)   The effects of experimental variations on problem solving in the rat. *J. Comp. Psychol.*, 45, 313–320.

Ingalls, T. H. (1950)   Anoxia as a course of foetal death and congenital defects in the mouse. *Am. J. Dis. child.*, 80, 34–45.

Klebanov, D. (1948)   Hunger und Physiche Erreginge ab ovar und Keinshadigungen. *Geburtsh und Frauenheilk*, 812, 7–8.

Knobloch, H. & Pasamanick, B. (1959a)   The syndrome of minimal cerebral damage in infancy *J.A.M.A.*, 170, 1384–1387.

Knobloch, H. & Pasamanick, B. (1959b)   Geographic and seasonal variations in birth rates. *Pub. Health Report.*, 74, 4, 285–289.

Kulka, A., Fry, C. & Goldstein, F. J. (1960)   Kinaesthetic needs in infancy. *Amer. J. Ortho. psychiat.*, 30, 306–314.

Liddicoat, R. (1968)   The effects of maternal antenatal decompression treatment on infant mental development. *S. A. Tydskrif vir Geneesekunde*, March 2nd, 203–211.

Lilienfeld, D. & Abraham, M. (1953) *Mass Study of reproductive wastage in prematurity congenital malformation.* New York: Assoc. for the aid of crippled children.

Lilienfeld, A. M., Pasamanick, B. & Rogers, M. (1955) Relationships between pregnancy experience and the development of certain neuropsychiatric disorders in childhood. *Am. J. Public Health,* 45, 637–643.

Melzack, R. (1968) A neuropsychological approach to heredity—environment. In G. Newton & S. Levine (Eds.) *Early experience and behaviour.* Springfield: Thomas.

Murphy, D. P. (1948) *Congenital malformations.* Philadelphia: Lippincott.

Newton G. & Levine, S. (Eds.) (1968) *Early experience and behaviour.* Springfield: Thomas.

Perlstein, M. A. (1952) Infantile cerebral palsy. Classifications and clinical correlations. *J. Am. Med. Assoc.,* 149, 30–34.

Perlstein, M. A. & Hood (1954) Infantile spastic hemiplegia. *Paediatrics,* 14, 436–441.

Perlstein, M. A. (1961) Epidemiological studies of the complications of pregnancy and birth. In G. Caplan (Ed.) *Prevention of mental disorders in children.* New York: Basic Books.

Potter, E. (1952) *Pathology of the foetus and the newborn.* Chicago: Year Book Pub. Inc.

Rogers, M., Lilienfeld, A. M. & Pasamanick, B. (1955) Prenatal and paranatal factors in the development of childhood behaviour disorders. *Acta Psychiat. et Neur. Scand.,* Supplement No. 102.

Schaffer, H. R. (1965) Changes in developmental quotient under two conditions of maternal separation. *Brit. J. Soc. Clin. Psych.* 4, 39–46.

Schaffer, H. R. (1966) Activity level as a constitutional determinant of infantile reaction to deprivation. *Child Dev.,* 37, 3, 596–602.

Schaffer, F. R. & Emerson, P. E. (1968) The effects of experimentally administered stimulation on the developmental quotients of children. *Brit. J. Soc. Clin. Psychol.* 7, 61–67.

Schulz, D. P. (1965) *Sensory restriction.* New York: Academic Press.

Scott-Russell, C. (1969) Another hazard of smoking. *New Scientist,* 9 Jan.

Smithells, R. W. & Morgan, D. H. (1970) Transmission of drugs by the placenta and breasts. *Prac.,* 204, 14–19.

Spitz, R. A. (1958) Quoted by Lebovice in *Review of Research in deprivation of maternal care.* W.H.O. Public Health Paper, 16, 82.

Strauss, A. A. & Kephart, N. C. (1955) *Psychopathology and education of the brain-injured child.* New York: Grune & Stratton.

Stott, D. H. (1957) Physical and mental handicaps following a disturbed pregnancy. *Lancet,* 18 May, 1006–1012

Stott, D. H. (1962) Mongolism related to early shock in pregnancy. Proceedings of the London conference on the Scientific study of Mental Deficiency. Dagenham: May & Baker.

Stott, D. H. (1966)   A general test of motor impairment for children. *Dev. Med. & Child Neur.*, 8, 523–531.

Walton, J. J., Ellis, E. & Court, S. D. M. (1962)   Clumsy children, developmental apraxia and agnosia. *Brain*, 85, 603.

Weiner, A. (1946)   Preventative aspects of rhesus incompatibility. *New York State Health News*, 26, 9–14.

Whiting, H. T. A., Johnson, G. F. & Page, M. (1969a)   The Gibson Spiral Maze as a possible screening device for minimal brain damage. *Brit. J. Soc. Clin. Psychol.*, 8, 164–168.

Whiting, H. T. A., Clarke, T. A. & Morris, P. R. (1969b)   A clinical validation of the Stott Test of motor impairment. *Brit. J. Soc. Clin. Psychol.*, 8, 270–274.

Whiting, H. T. A., Davies, J. G., Gibson, J. M., Lumley, R., Sutcliffe, R. S. E. & Morris, P. R. (1970)   Motor impairment in an approved school population. Unpublished paper, Physical Education Dept., Leeds University.

Workany, J. (1950)   Congenital malformations. In Mitchell Nelson (Ed.) *Textbook of paediatrics*. Philadelphia: Saunders.

Zeulzer, W. W. (1950)   Kernicterus. Aetiological study based on analysis of 55 cases. *Paediatrics*, 6, 452–474.

CHAPTER 3

Motor Impairment and Intellectual Development

> *Body and mind are never independent. Such subdivision*
> *is entirely arbitrary and unfounded. Although much re-*
> *mains to be learned about the brain and CNS, neurolo-*
> *gists in general, agree that the idea of two lives, somatic*
> *and psychic, has outlived its usefulness. Thus, the psycho-*
> *somatic concept of medicine recognises this fact of integra-*
> *tion and acknowledges its significance.*
>
> (Ismail & Gruber, 1967)

In discussing the skill model in Chapter 1, attention was drawn
to the many subsystems involved in human performance in
addition to the motor mechanisms themselves. Particular
emphasis was placed on the ability of the model to accommodate
skills of many kinds which collectively can be classified as
perceptual-motor. On this basis alone, it would not be surprising to find that deficiencies in any of the subsystems resulted
not only in impairment in motor behaviour but also in behaviour of a more cognitive kind.

While many instances of children suffering deficits in intellectual, motor and social development can be found, the *generality*
of such a finding would be difficult to establish. This reflects
not only a difficulty in assessment, but the fact that a child
who shows evidence of motor impairment and who is of average
ability in terms of intelligence might be deemed to be impaired
only in those subsystems primarily related to motor skill
performance. What is often missed here, is that the potential
ability of the child in terms of intelligence might be well above
the standard which he currently exhibits. A more serious
difficulty may also arise in that when a motor-impaired child is
apparently adapting well (i.e. showing a reasonable level of

73

intellectual and social behaviour) his deficit on the motor side which may reflect a retardation in all areas of development may not be appreciated. At more extreme levels, where children show marked intellectual deficit (E.S.N. children)—the focusing of attention on such deficit may lead those concerned with compensatory education to appreciate that such retardation may extend to the motor and often the social field as was made apparent in the case-histories previously reported (pages 37–39).

Motor ability and early cognitive development

The significance of movement for early cognitive development is receiving new emphasis although it is by no means a novel relationship. As long ago as 1912, Welton had this to say:

> . . . the need of children for bodily activity is being increasingly acknowledged in practice, though slowly and somewhat grudgingly. Despite all the indications of nature, children of five years and upwards are still made to sit for long hours in desks mainly looking and listening. Public opinion is satisfied if a few minutes daily be spent in the playground and if, two or three times a week the children be put through some form of bodily drill. Even these deliverances from the desk are, however, advocated purely from a physical standpoint. . . . Modern knowledge enables us to go further and to affirm that the relation between body and mind is so intimate and constant that the intelligence is dwarfed whenever the demand for bodily activity is not met.

Because of the developments which have occurred over the past 50 or so years, the greater part of the above critique would not be justified—at least in the United Kingdom. At the same time, it must be asked to what extent educationalists pay more than lip service to the concept elaborated in Welton's last sentence? If this statement of 'psychophysical monism' is accepted, it should certainly be one of the central propositions of any educational system particularly in relation to early development. To what extent have the past 50 years seen not only an appreciation of this idea, but the instituting of educational procedures designed specifically to elaborate upon its implications? To what extent is movement experience in the home and early school fostered in the belief that without sufficient and appropriate movement experience, cognitive development is retarded?

Some of the evidence for the effects of movement experience on early cognitive development have already been discussed in relation to 'deprivation' (pages 61–63) and the reader is referred back to this evidence.

Piaget (1953) in particular has described a sensori-motor period related to the development of intelligence in children. This period begins with reflex actions and continues until language and symbolism begin to make their appearance. In essence, the implication of this stage of development is that education through the medium of movement precedes verbal education and can therefore be considered to be fundamental. In Piaget's terms, restricted experience—including restricted movement experience—would affect the development of 'schemata' or in Hebb's (1949) terms the development of 'cell-assemblies' on which later intellectual development depends.

Piaget's position in this respect has been summarised by Tamburrini (1968):

> Piaget would say that we cannot really speak of 'mind' in relation to the new-born infant. What he brings into the world are certain reflexes, and he himself gradually constructs his mind. By means of these ready made reflexes, for example of sucking when something comes into contact with his lips, of grasping when something comes into his hands and of looking when something comes into his direct visual field, the child reacts to the environment when stimulated. From birth the child begins to exercise these reflexes, but within a very short time they show variations and modifications; he begins to discriminate . . . they become active rather than passive; the result is searching behaviour . . . and at this point they (the reflexes) have been replaced by learned behaviour patterns: or what Piaget calls Schemas. . . . In Piaget's words, the child constructs reality.

That a tacit link at least is accepted between motor and intellectual performance is reflected in a review of Binet-type intelligence scales. Many items can be found which involve motor performance although primarily of fine motor skills. Intelligence tests such as the W.I.S.C. (Wechsler, 1949) enable the assessment of both a verbal and a *performance* IQ. The earlier it is wished to assess a child's intelligence level, the more recourse there is to tests involving motor skills. At the very earliest level, the tester is restricted even further to the assessment of primitive reflexes such as those involved in the methods of St. Ann Dargaisses. The *prognostic* value of such early assessments is not particularly good. Table 2 for example (Carmichael, 1952) shows retest correlations at 3-year intervals from two separate studies suggesting the trends to be expected.

TABLE 2

Test-retest correlations at 3-year intervals

	Elbert & Simmons (1945)	Honzik et al. (1948)
Age 2 by 5	—	0·32 ±0·06 P.E.
3 by 6	0·56 ±0·04 P.E.	0·57 ±0·03
4 by 7	0·55 ±0·04	0·59 ±0·03
5 by 8	0·70 ±0·03	0·70 ±0·02
7 by 10	0·76 ±0·02	0·78 ±0·02
9 by 12 or 13	—	0·85 ±0·01

Farmer's (1927) comments may give part of the explanation of the decreasing value of tests of motor ability as assessors of mental ability:

Among young children fairly high correlations have been found between certain motor tests and tests of intelligence but these intercorrelations tend to become smaller as the age of the child increases. The explanation of this appears to be that motor tests for young children are not really tests of motor capacity but of intelligence, since with a partially developed intelligence it is only the really intelligent children who understand what is required of them in a motor test. As specialisation increases this ceases to be the case, and the fact that motor tests no longer correlate with intelligence shows that they have ceased to be tests of intelligence, and have become as they were intended, tests of motor capacity.

It is interesting to note the way in which many developmental psychologists categorise tests giving the impression of independent modes of development. Gesell (1928) for example has developmental scales for:

motor development
language development
adaptive behaviour
personal-social adjustment

but also states that:

> during infancy the mind and body follow a course primordially determined.

Griffiths (1954) in assessing the abilities of babies uses the following categorisation:

locomotor development
personal-social adjustment
hearing and speech
hand-eye coordination
performance (reasoning, intelligence, manipulation)

and in a similar way, Buhler (1935) suggests:

sensory reception
bodily movements
social behaviour
learning
manipulation of materials
mental production

Hurlock (1949) on the other hand, does not divide the items into classified groups but rather sets out behaviour patterns which might be expected at six-monthly intervals.

e.g. at the six month level:
1. Recognises name.
   call baby's name and several others all in the same tone.
   Pass if recognises name, turns head and smiles.
2. Lifts cup.
   Sitting position in mother's lap near table.
   Throw 1 inch cube on table. While child is looking, cover it with a cup. Draw cup to within reach handle of cup to the right. *Pass* if he lifts the cup. He need not remove or pick up the cube.
3. Hitting stationary object.
   Sitting on lap. Give him rattle to hold. Dangle small toy on 5″ string close enough to hit it with the rattle.
   Pass if he hits it with rattle or attempts to seriously.
4. Pulls to sitting position.
   Examiner stands at the foot of crib and offers thumbs.
   Allow him with this support to pull to sitting. Do not pull, but raise hands gradually as he pulls.
   Pass if he arrives in sitting position.

These items all require motor behaviour, although some authorities would probably classify number 1 as personal-social, number 2 as learning or adaptive, number 3 as hand-eye coordination leaving number 4 in the bodily movement category. Hurlock's tests generally appear to contain a bias towards motor behaviour. The 18-month level includes items such as drinking several mouthfuls without a pause and being able to get off a box 6 inches high other than by falling off. The test at 2 years includes imitation of simple movements such as lifting both arms above the head, clapping, putting hands on head, and circling hands round one another.

Hurlock considers muscle and intelligence to be closely related. Morgan & King (1966) on the other hand imply that the development of reflexes and motor abilities is *just* a matter of maturation and that speed of development is not necessarily an indication of intelligence. Griffiths (1954) further suggests that all one can measure in the young infant is a 'general quotient' but feels that:

> the rate of progression in early infancy is
> relevant in assessing the mental level.

In contradiction to some of the workers quoted, Illingworth (1963) considers gross motor development to be the least important field for the assessment of intelligence.

Motor and mental ability

The possibility of a significant positive relationship between motor and mental performance was recognised by early workers in the intelligence field even prior to Welton (1912) but it would appear that there were many misconceptions. Procedures involving such variables as reaction time and physical measures were typical of the approach of Galton as long ago as 1884 and while at the time such tests were not particularly productive they were the forerunners of present-day developments.

Bagley (1900) conducted one of the earlier studies into the relationship between motor and mental ability. His study showed a general inverse relation. Those who were intellectually brighter and had a faster reaction time being as a rule deficient in motor ability while those who were best developed physically, who were the strongest and who had developed motor control to the greatest extent were generally deficient in mental ability. Numerous individual exceptions were, however, apparent and the validity of this study might be questioned.

Wisler (1901) carried out an interesting study into the correlation between mental and physical performances. The following tests were made upon 60–70 freshmen at Columbia College:

Length and breadth of head, strength of hands, fatigue, eyesight and colour vision, hearing and perception of pitch, perception of weight, sensation areas, sensitiveness to pain, perception of size, colour preference, reaction time, rate of perception, naming colours, rate of movement, perception of time, association, imagery and memory together with data on stature and weight, personal habits and health. Wisler's criterion of mental ability was in fact class-standing rather than on some formal test such as the later developed IQ tests. In general, intercorrelations between the tests were very low. Wisler's comments in his discussion on the concept of abilities:

> What constitutes mental ability? . . . all tests in this series have little interdependence. . . . It is plain that if we accept the conclusion of this research as final, an individual must be regarded as the algebraic sum of a vast array of small abilities of almost equal probability, the resulting combination conforming to the laws of chance.

There are numerous research reports in the literature into the relationship between motor and mental ability. At this stage, there is little point in discussing these in detail as results are in the main conflicting. The following are typical studies:

Garfield (1923) quotes correlations from 0·01 to 0·12 for adults between motor ability and intelligence. Brace (1932) reports correlations between 0 and 0·2 between mental ability and physical ability. Johnson (1932) found a correlation of 0·49 for college men and 0·13 for junior high school boys on tests of intelligence and physical skill. McCloy (1934) reports a correlation of $-0·125$ between motor ability and IQ. Ray (1940) found correlations between mental ability and physical ability ranging from $-0·11$ to $+0·27$; between mental ability and physical achievement from 0·03 to 0·17; between mental achievement and physical ability from 0·09 to 0·24 and between mental achievement and physical achievement from 0·07 to 0·76. Espenchade (1940) tested 165 adolescent boys and girls on a series of gross motor measures. The results for the boys showed a positive significant relationship between motor performance and chronological, emotional and physical maturity. The girls' motor performances correlated very low with all measures of physical growth.

The confusion that exists and the disagreement as to the precise relationship pertaining between motor and mental ability is amply borne out by the selection of results quoted above. It seems probable that the diversity of motor demands in different tests and the difficulties implicit in tests for a general factor of motor ability are perhaps the main reasons for the conflicting results.

In a comprehensive overview of physical parameters and intellectual performance Ismail & Gruber (1967) summarise:

> After reviewing the literature one would be likely to conclude that the relationships between intellectual performance and items measuring physical growth, strength, speed and power were low and in some cases non-existent. These findings were consistent in both sexes and were presented by many researchers including the authors of this book. . . . It was shown that motor performance scores improve with age and grade level. In addition, early physical maturing boys have a distinct advantage in tests of motor performance. It is also noted that the relationship between physical fitness and intellectual achievement is not firmly established.

Ismail & Gruber noting an absence in the literature of work concerned with investigating the relationship between items measuring a 'more innate motor aptitude domain'—namely balance, coordination and kinethesis—carried out an extensive factor analytic study designed to clarify this issue. A review of their findings suggests that:

> 1. Growth in general is not associated with intelligence except in the case of low achievers.
> 2. Speed, power, strength and accuracy are generally not related to intelligence.
> 3. Coordination is not related to intelligence except in the case of medium achievers.
> 4. Balance and kinesthesis are not related to intelligence.
> 5. In general, growth items are related to academic achievement.

6. Speed, power, strength and accuracy correlated differently among the three levels of achievers.
7. Coordination is related to academic achievement.
8. Balance and kinesthesis are not related to academic achievement.

Subsidiary analyses and factor patterns together with predictive batteries are reported but are beyond the scope of the present discussion.

Motor ability and mental subnormality

There would appear to be more agreement amongst workers in the field, of a significant positive relationship between motor and mental ability if the complete range of mental ability is taken into consideration. Malpass (1963) in a review of relevant literature and research on this topic, investigated such a relationship in normal and mentally retarded subjects. He concluded from his study that the mentally retarded children tended to demonstrate less motor competence and skills than normals of the same age and sex. This finding generalised across both precise manipulative skills and more complex gross motor coordination tasks. If Malpass's review of studies together with his own findings are accepted, it seems likely that motor impairment or motor disability is more likely to be found in a population of below average IQ.

Support for this contention is provided by Fish (1961) who investigated the possibility of a significant relationship between a disturbance in early motor development and the level of later intellectual functioning. She noted that in school-age children, if the disturbance was sufficiently severe as to interfere with intellectual functioning, then it also tended to be associated with a derangement of the motor and perceptual functions. Fish points out that the severity of the impairment depends on the timing and duration of early neural disturbance and on environmental factors.

In a similar vein, Malpass (1959) reports that more than 45% of his retarded adolescents were not walking by the sixteenth postpartum month and 20% did not walk until after 26 months of age.

The Lincoln–Oseretzky test (from which the Stott (1966) test of motor impairment originally derived) has been used by a number of investigators seeking the nature of the relationship between impaired motor and intellectual performance (Sloan, 1950; Rabin, 1957; Di Stefano *et al.*, 1958; Malpass, 1960).

Sloan (1950) reported a significant relationship between scores made by institution defectives on his 1948 adaptation of the Oseretzky test and the Stanford–Binet (1937) intelligence test. The group tested, however, was only twenty in number. Sloan comments:

> Within the limitations of this study we may conclude that motor proficiency is related to intelligence. Motor proficiency is not a distinct aspect of functioning which can be isolated from general behaviour, but is, rather, another aspect of the total functioning which cannot be isolated from general behaviour of the organism. It would appear that an adequate evaluation of adaptive capacity should include not only estimates of intelligence but of motor proficiency and social maturity as well.

Rabin (1957) found no significant relationship between scores on the Lincoln–Oseretzky and Stanford–Binet scales. He attributed the lack of such a relationship to an uncontrolled 'examiner institutional' variable.

Di Stefano *et al.* (1958) report correlations of 0·40 and 0·58 for similar tests on institutionalised boys and girls respectively.

Malpass (1960) again on institutionalised boys and girls respectively reports correlations of 0·48 and 0·27 between the Lincoln–Oseretzky and the Wechsler Intelligence Scale for children. He also reports correlations of 0·34 and 0·75 for non-institutionalised boys and girls. The high correlation reported for the girls was attributed to a chance sampling factor as there were only twenty-three in the sample.

A further study utilising factor-analytic techniques and including the Stott (1966) test of motor impairment (page 171) as one of the tests in the battery utilised is of interest. In this study, Whiting *et al.* (1969b) gave a battery of tests to a sample (population of two E.S.N. schools) of fifty E.S.N. children between the ages of 10 and 11 years (Mean Terman–Merrill IQ 68·7). The tests covered areas concerned with manual dexterity (Minnesota Rate of Manipulation Test); field dependence/independence in Witkin's (1962) terms (Embedded Figures Test); personality in perceptual-motor terms (Gibson (1965) spiral maze); brain-damage (Memory for designs test—

Graham & Kendall (1960)); Motor Impersistence-Test—Garfield (1966); Sophistication of Body Concept (Draw-a-man Test); Motor Impairment (Stott, 1966 test)—Stott I (5 item) and Stott II (3 item) together with the parameters IQ, age, height and weight. The inter-correlations between the tests were subjected to a principal components analysis (Table 3). Of particular interest in the present context, is Factor 1 which can be identified as a more general factor of impairment accounting for 30% of the variance and reflecting the relationship which exists between a low IQ and a high motor impairment score within *this population*. It is also interesting to note the high loadings on this factor of the two tests purporting to assess brain damage (Memory for designs test: Test of motor impersistence).

TABLE 3

Principal Components Analysis for a population of
10–11-year-old E.S.N. schoolchildren

Test	I	II	III	IV	V	VI
			Components			
1. IQ	−58	36	11	14	−25	49
2. Memory for des.	59	−27	−49	−24	—	—
3. Manual dexterity	74	−11	−19	—	−23	15
4. Motor Impersist.	74	−32	−22	—	—	—
5. Stott I	94	—	−13	12	—	—
6. Stott II	95	11	—	10	—	—
7. Draw-a-man	17	11	−91	−24	—	—
8. Embedded Figs.	29	−17	−59	—	−11	67
9. Spiral Maze-Time	14	89	−15	−14	—	—
10. Spiral Maze-error	−43	−73	−22	13	—	16
11. Age	—	—	—	14	95	—
12. Height	—	—	16	83	—	26
13. Weight	—	−13	−17	82	—	−40
% Variance	29·9	13·5	13·0	12·0	8·3	7·9

Decimal points and loadings between ± 0·1 omitted.

The 'ability' concept

Although the possibility of a *general* impairment embracing all forms of skilled behaviour has been raised a number of times—particularly in relation to E.S.N. children—the *usefulness* of a concept such as *general* ability in the motor or mental field is open to question. The trend in analyses and in compensatory education programmes is rather to focus attention on basic abilities which enter into a wide range of different activities. In the analysis of intelligence for example, Vernon (1950) summarises the major findings as suggesting factors of verbal, spatial, numerical, mathematical and manual ability. Since these factors of intelligence are not independent, it is possible to account for their intercorrelations in terms of a more general factor. Thus, it is largely a question of emphasis and usefulness whether particular workers choose to focus on the more general ability factor or on abilities of a less general nature.

In a recent review of the work in the motor performance field, Fleishman (1967) suggests that if a person performs at a consistently high level in a selection of different tasks and not particularly well in another selection, it indicates that there is a common process involved in performing the one series of tasks. Abilities are those mechanisms which account for the observed consistencies. He suggests further that they should be regarded as more general traits of the individual which have been inferred from certain consistencies on certain kinds of tasks. Fleishman differentiates between 'ability' and 'skill'. The latter represents the level of proficiency on a specific task or limited group of tasks. Abilities enter into and are necessary for the performance of skills. Certain abilities are more basic in the sense that they are related to performance on diverse tasks.

From a practical point of view, the implication of this kind of work is that skilled performance depends upon abilities which are present before embarking on the task together with habits and subskills which are peculiar to and acquired within the task itself. The idea that basic abilities place limits on later skill proficiency is of fundamental concern in relation to motor and intellectual impairment. If in fact brain damage is present, or children have undergone sensory/perceptual deprivation or a combination of the two, it might reasonably be supposed that the possibility of their developing the appropriate abilities to a normal level will be severely limited and subsequent skill behaviour will be affected. It also draws attention once again to the fundamental importance of early movement experience on which many of these basic abilities depend. Thus, it would appear that early movement experience of a diverse kind contributes towards the development of abilities which enter into the performance of all kinds of skills at some later stage. Such experience will include reflex movement patterns and the practice of less complex skills. A reciprocal relationship would seem to exist. The practice of reflex reactions and low level skills leads to the building up of abilities and such abilities contribute towards the acquisition of more complex skills at some later stage. Such abilities may be primarily genetically determined (as in colour-blindness) or primary experiential (as in aiming).

Fleishman (1967) identified the following abilities by factor analytic techniques:

1. Control precision
2. Multi-limb coordination
3. Response orientation
4. Reaction time
5. Speed of movement
6. Rate control
7. Manual dexterity
8. Finger dexterity
9. Arm-hand steadiness
10. Wrist-finger speed
11. Aiming

In some skills, abilities which contribute to performance early in the learning process are not necessarily the same abilities which contribute to later performance. This is reflected in the following statement and should be a sobering thought to those 'experts' in particular skill areas who attempt to teach the beginner on the basis of what the expert performer is known or assumed to do:

> The ability-skill paradigm and the experimental results based on it is consistent with an information processing model of human learning. Abilities can be thought of as 'capacities for utilising different kinds of information'. Thus, individuals who are especially good at using certain types of spatial information, make rapid progress in the early stages of learning certain kinds of motor tasks, while individuals sensitive to proprioceptive cues do better in tasks requiring precise motor control.

It is not entirely clear what relationship these abilities have to what he variously terms, 'spatial orientation' or 'spatial visualisation', these being referred to as 'general abilities'.

Although Fleishman does not raise the point in his review, it is worth asking whether or not the ability to utilise spatial or proprioceptive information is in some ways different or more basic than other abilities listed? He does, however, point out that some abilities may be required in most skills. These are the abilities associated with spatial-temporal patterning and those abilities that are related to the organisation of responses. Speculation about the reasons underlying such individual differences might be worth while. The most useful link in this respect is that made by Wober (1965) on cross-cultural differences in reliance on particular forms of information processing which is discussed further in Chapter 5 (page 128).

On the question of the specificity or generality of the abilities required to perform psychomotor tasks, Yates (1968) suggests that the long line of experimental results stretching from Seashore (1940) to Fleishman (1954) produce agreement on the fact that:

> although a general factor of psychomotor ability cannot be doubted its importance has generally been rejected

a comment which was raised at the beginning of this section. The solution preferred has been that which rests upon relatively independent group factors, clusters of these group factors entering into the performance of different skills. Mention should perhaps be made of the fact that the majority of the factorial studies in this area have been carried out with highly selected groups for special purposes. For example, many of Fleishman's most sophisticated studies have been carried out in an attempt to devise selection tests for highly skilled positions in the American forces. This is not to deny the usefulness of the studies, but to merit caution in extrapolating to other populations.

Again, the abilities isolated by different workers are not necessarily definitive. They are dependent, as are the majority of these types of study upon the nature of the test batteries used. These have differed widely from study to study.

If the ideas discussed so far are accepted, it follows that the individual who has a great many highly developed basic abilities can become proficient at a great variety of specific tasks. The failure of many investigations to isolate a *general* motor ability factor accounting for a *major* portion of the variance may reflect the fact that the all-round development of abilities is still severely limited, or that it is usually only possible for a limited range of experience to be presented to the majority of children. This should not lead educationalists to suppose that more enriched environments or different methods of child-rearing might not lead to superior development. Too little research at the present time has gone into the effect of enriched early experience or to the teaching of particular skills at particular age levels. Concepts of 'age of readiness' and 'critical periods' are bandied about with little firm evidence in the field of *human* behaviour. As Connolly (1968) suggests, failure or great difficulty on the part of a child to learn a given response has frequently been accounted for in terms of the child's not being ready or not being able to learn the response at the time whereas more concern should be centred around the efficiency of the teaching techniques adopted.

The ongoing work on abilities has a number of implications for the study of motor impairment. Concern has not rested merely at screening off those children who are impaired by some acceptable criterion (although devices of this nature might be useful as a first procedure—Whiting *et al.* (1969b)) but from the original work of Oseretzky (1923) through the various revisions (Yarmolenko, 1933; Doll, 1946; Sloan, 1948, 1955) down to the work of Stott (1966) there has been an attempt to isolate the factors underlying the *particular* deficiency(ies) of impaired children. Few of the studies indicate any serious attempt to map out a hierarchy of abilities. One recent study is perhaps an exception—that of Sapir *et al.* (1967). The Sapir developmental scale was designed to indicate the deficiencies of children judged as having 'minimum cerebral dysfunction'. From eighteen children identified on this criterion, Table 4 (overleaf) shows the different areas of impairment coupled with the frequency with which each area (ability?) was involved.

Sapir *et al.* suggest that specific compensatory education should be tailored to the needs of each child and further point out that the individual patterns of deficit differ so widely that differential diagnosis is an essential pre-requisite for appropriate remedial work. This approach is reflected by many workers in the field. A diagnostic profile is built up of the child's deficiencies and then a programme arranged to assist in each of the areas. The results quoted in Table 4 indicate that certain of the areas of deficit are more common than others

TABLE 4

Area tested	No. of times area involved in deficiency pattern ($N = 18$)
Visual discrimination	5
Visual memory	5
Auditory design	9
Auditory memory	6
Visual motor	11
Directionality/laterality	13
Spatial relations	11
Body schema	5
Language	5
Orientation	6

(directionality/laterality, spatial relations, visual motor) although the number in the sample from which these were derived was relatively small. If this turns out to be a more general finding attention should be concentrated on these areas. It would also appear to be necessary, following on from Fleishman's work to discover the extent to which proficiency in these areas is involved in the performance of the widest range of everyday skills required by children from a number of socio-economic groupings. These abilities might then be developed in pre-school and 'headstart' programmes. To some extent this approach is already utilised by different workers. The programmes developed by Kephart (1960), Chaney & Kephart (1968), Doman & Delacato (1967), Bobath (1966) and Radin & Sonquist (1968) emphasise the importance of such abilities and particularly the awareness of laterality and directionality in relation to the individual's own body.

Spatial ability

It is not possible within the confines of a short chapter to deal in any detail with all the particular abilities which have been isolated. There would, however, seem to be some merit in focusing attention on spatial ability which has been shown to be a major group factor (more general) in both motor and mental performance. Vernon (1950) for example with others has shown a spatial factor to be important in a multi-factorial analysis of intelligence and Smith (1964) has indicated the important relationship it bears to academic achievement. In an earlier study (Smith, 1954) the latter worker showed that a test of spatial ability was the best single predictor of success for the selection of boys for a technical course and other tests did little to add to the predictive value. A number of investigators have noted the correlation between various disorders of spatial disability and impairment (Caldwell, 1956; Hebb, 1939; Abercrombie, 1964; Cruickshank *et al.*, 1957; Brenner *et al.*, 1967). Spatial tests in one form or another are quite common in test batteries for motor impairment. Evidence is available which suggests that certain spatial tests are particularly sensitive to motor impairment and the effects of brain damage. In particular, the Porteus mazes (Porteus, 1959), various forms of memory-for-designs tests (Graham & Kendall, 1946; Siskind, 1966), the trail-maker test (Reitan, 1958) and the Gibson Spiral Maze (Gibson, 1964).

Whiting *et al.* (1969b) used the Gibson Spiral Maze as a possible screening device for motor impairment in an E.S.N. population. The relative effectiveness of the 'slow and careless' quadrant as a screen as compared with the Stott Test of motor impairment and two tests of brain damage [Memory for Designs Test (Graham & Kendall (1960)) and Motor Impersistence Test (Garfield (1964))] is indicated in Table 5 & Figure 6. Attention is drawn to the high percentage of brain-damaged children (assuming the validity of the tests selected) within this E.S.N. population.

TABLE 5

Screening efficiency: E.S.N. group

Section	Spiral Maze	M.F.D. Critical	Motor impersistence (2 +failures)	Stott Test failures
Slow and careless	15	12	13	11
Quick and careless	9	5	6	3
Quick and accurate	18	2	2	1
Slow and accurate	8	3	3	2
n =	50	22	24	17

In a further study on an approved school population of sixty-two boys between the ages of 11 years and 14 years, Whiting *et al.* (1970) included the Gibson Spiral Maze as part of a larger test battery. The results of the screening efficiency for this population are given in a similar way in Table 6 and Figure 7.

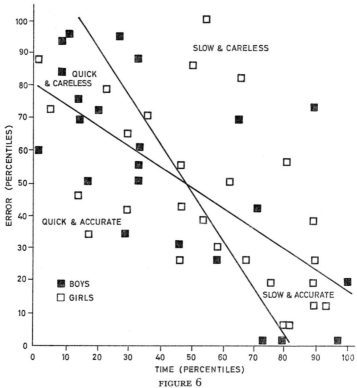

FIGURE 6

Scatter plot for the E.S.N. group. ■, boys; □, girls

It will be noted that in this population very few children were screened off as being brain-damaged. The evidence available from case records was more suggestive of multiple-causality in which deprivation in one form or another figured highly.

TABLE 6

Screening efficiency: approved school population

Quadrant	Spiral Maze N	M.F.D. Borderline N	Critical N	Motor impersistence failures N	Stott test N
Slow and careless	19	4	3	0	9
Quick and careless	14	5	3	0	3
Quick and accurate	18	2	1	1	2
Slow and accurate	9	3	1	0	2
Total	60	14	8	1	16

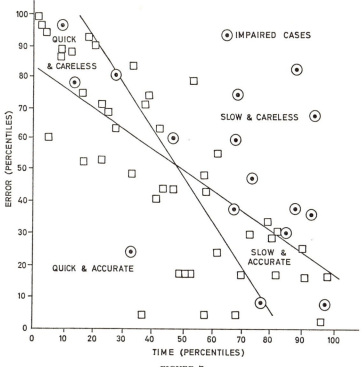

FIGURE 7

Scatter plot for the Approved School group

Spatial ability would appear to be a generic term for a particular grouping of abilities which fall mainly into three areas (Michael *et al.*, 1957)—spatial relation and orientation; spatial visualisation and kinesthetic imagery. Thurstone (1950) suggests further that visual orientation in space relates to three factors:

1. Ability to recognise the identity of an object when it is seen from different angles.
2. Ability to imagine the movement or internal displacement among parts of a configuration.
3. Ability to think about spatial relations in which the body orientation of the observer is an essential part of the problem.

There is an overlap here with French's (1951) suggestion that spatial ability involves:

1. The ability to perceive spatial patterns accurately and to compare them with each other.
2. The ability to be unconfused by varying orientations in which a spatial pattern may be presented.
3. The ability to comprehend imaginary movement in three dimensional space or manipulate objects in imagination.

With the above elaboration of the area covered, it is not difficult to understand the important role played by such an ability in a wide range of skilled behaviour. Having therefore established the importance of spatial ability, it is worth looking at the way in which such an ability is developed in the hope that it will shed some light on the impairment problem.

A lead is given by Fleishman (1967) in the reference already quoted (page 85) where he refers to abilities as being means of dealing with different kinds of information. This suggestion provides a link between 'abilities' and the 'analyser' concept of Deutsch (1960) and Sutherland (1959); the 'filter' theory of Broadbent (1958), Treisman (1969) and Norman (1968) and Piaget's (1952) concept of 'schemata'. Although in some ways disparate, all these approaches have in common a model incorporating some kind of 'template' which may be used to identify inputs and determine outputs of the C.N.S.

The evidence for the existence of such 'templates' or 'analysers' and their genetic and experimental origins is closely interrelated. In view of this, it may be appropriate to consider the way in which a number of differently oriented investigators have seen this relationship and indicate the relevance of such work to the study and treatment of motor impairment.

Hershenson (1967) suggests that the first consideration is an analysis of the newborn infant's ability to respond to form. If the newborn infant can perceive form then the developmental problem is one of modification and improvement rather than construction. The question posed therefore, is the nature of the possible antecedents to 'form perception processes' which would mediate responses to stimuli containing form but which could not be labelled form perception? Hebb (1949), Sackett (1963) and Dodwell (1964) suggest that there is a system of 'primary elements' or invariance detectors which combine to form functionally autonomous structures. Data from experiments carried out by Kessen et al. (1965) provides evidence for the existence of invariance detectors in human newborns. The type of experiment carried out is best illustrated from the work of Salapatek & Kessen (1966). In this investigation twenty awake, alert newborns, under eight days old, were placed in a situation where they viewed first an homogeneous black field and later a large, solid central triangle. In the first situation, the visual scanning of the infants was widely dispersed with the greater dispersion in the horizontal rather than the vertical dimensions. In the case of the triangle, the dispersal of the scanning was reduced. The infant responded to only part of the figure and the ocular orientations were not distributed haphazardly, over the triangle but were clustered at the vertices. One of the interpretations of the results is that the infants may respond to angles. This interpretation the authors suggest is congruent with the analyser theories of discrimination as suggested by Sutherland (1959), Deutsch (1960) and Dodwell (1964).

Fantz (1967) in reporting on his experiments which were concerned with the responses of newborn infants to various arrangements of schematic facial features claims that his results backed by the evidence of workers such as Hershenon *et al.* (1965) and Stechler (1964) showed

> that some degree of perception is unlearned in the neonate, whatever changes and improvements occur subsequently

A failure to appreciate the presence of abilities of selective attention/perception in the newborn has been unfortunate. As Lipsitt (1969) points out:

> It has been implicitly assumed that intellectual endowment is genetically determined and essentially constant; proper attention has not been paid to the behavioural consequences of experimental precursors. These attitudes and assumptions have almost pre-empted the search for, and discovery of the special capacity of infants to receive sensory stimulation in all modalities and to learn.

While evidence such as that quoted strongly supports the genetic basis of the analyser/ability mechanisms, it does not rule out the part played by subsequent experience or the effects of inter uterine development. Fantz refers to the evidence that experience affects this perception and concludes:

Just as initial visual preferences reveal the unlearned beginnings of perception and visual attention, subsequent changes reveal effects of age and experience.

The effect of prolonged visual deprivation for example interferes with what appears to be some form of sequential build up of analysers and therefore alters the subsequent effects of visual experience. Walk & Gibson (1961) illustrate a case where infants kept in darkness for less than a month followed by several days of unrestricted experience avoided walking on glass over an apparent 30 inch spatial drop. Longer deprived infants required many days of experience, or else within the confines of the experimental situation never did avoid the cliff side of the apparatus.

In connection with the development of 'schemata' Piaget indicates that the sensori motor systems regularly involved in an infant's interaction with his environmental circumstances develop much more rapidly than they would if not used. According to Piaget (1952):

Use is the alignment of schema.

In commenting upon the coordination of grasping and looking which appeared in his son at three months, and in his daughter at 6 months he states:

However, nothing justifies us in considering Jacquelin retarded . . . the explanation is simple. Jacquelin born January 9th and spending her days outdoors on a balcony, was much less active in the beginning than Laurent, born in May. Furthermore, and by virtue of this fact, I made fewer experiments on her during the first months, whereas I was constantly busy with Laurent.

Much recent research supports Piaget's observations. Two examples may be taken as typical of the many investigations carried out in this area. Greenberg, Uzgiris & Hunt (1968) conducted an experiment in which a stable pattern was suspended within view over the cribs of home reared infants from the age of 5 weeks. This resulted in the appearance of a blink response considerably earlier than in a control group. White & Held (1966) demonstrated that the opportunity to look at objects hastened the development of visual accommodation upon which the blink response is based. They suggest that the development of attention is a function of circumstances.

There would also appear to be support for Hebb's (1949) suggestion that neural maturation and the development of brain structure and chemistry appear to be influenced appreciably by environmental encounters. In other words, even reflex systems decay without use. Investigations with animals (Weiskrantz, 1958; Lieberman, 1962) have shown that the absence of an opportunity to use the eyes to see light and patterns results in failure of the anatomical apparatus of the visual system to develop. There is also support for the other side of the picture, namely, that there is increased growth of central brain structures of rats developing in circumstances deliberately made extra complex (Altman & Das, 1964; Bennett et al., 1964).

Before leaving this area, the relationship between a genetic base and the effects of early experiences elaborated by White (1969) is worth reporting. This study involved 300 hospital-reared children who were observed for 3 hours per week for 6 months. The experimental group in this study, who were reared under conditions designed to increase the occurrence of certain forms of motility in sensorily enriched environments, produced markedly precocious visually directed reaching and heightened visual attentiveness.

A summary of the work outlined in relation to abilities and suggestions which might be appropriate in relation to motor impairment follows:

1. 'Spatial ability' with its dependence upon the development of appropriate 'analysers' has a genetic basis. From the point of motor impairment, this is a given determinant about which little can be done.
2. Interacting with the given genetic base is early experience. The tenor of the evidence presented indicates that the subsequent development of abilities may be markedly affected by the quality of this early experience. It may be argued that due to the very real difficulties of identifying impaired children below the age of 6 months means that when they are discovered it is rather late to effect any changes. Once again, much of this may be true. However, in a number of areas it is possible to identify children who may be impaired at a very early stage. It is fairly well established that various

forms of stress during pregnancy and difficulties during labour are very closely correlated with future impairment (Strauss & Kephart, 1955; Fairweather & Illsley, 1960; Corah et al., 1968; Stott, 1966). It should be possible in cases of difficulties in pregnancy to arrange for the child to be exposed, at a very early stage, to the type of visual stimulation on which the development of 'spatial ability' appears to rest.

3. Concerning the cases of impairment that are identified at a later stage of development the question arises, Is it possible to develop 'spatial ability'? A tentative answer is 'yes'. The type of evidence leading towards this affirmative answer is now discussed.

Reviewing the experimental work with mature individuals Gibson (1953) reported that practice resulted in improvement of the ability to discriminate in tasks involving visual space and the perception of depth and distance. In a more recent study, Gibson et al. (1962) have shown that the ability to discriminate letter-like forms in various dimensions improved with age and experience.

In considering the conditions necessary for the type of perceptual learning hypothesised, Gibson (1962) states:

> It may be that the child learns which varying dimensions are significant and which are not by simply looking repeatedly at many samples containing both varying and invariant features. The distinctive features are not taught but they are nevertheless learned.

It does appear that sheer repeated observation may facilitate discrimination.

One finding that has implications for the education of impaired children, emanates from an experiment conducted by Bijou & Baer (1963). They found that by using operant conditioning procedures they were able to shorten the normal developmental period delineated above by Gibson. Vernon (1957) reported that 5-five-year-old children were unable to distinguish mirror reversals, yet Bijou & Baer were able to train 5-year-olds to the level of flawless performance.

If the theoretical argument followed here is correct then it should be possible, by structuring the exposure to appropriate stimulation, to at least improve the ability in this area. This possibility is reflected in relation to African children by a study carried out by Poole (1969). The control group in this study was made up of eighteen spatially deprived African children. The experimental group of four children were given thirty-eight sessions spread over 8 weeks in which they were exposed to a spatial enrichment programme. The results of the two groups on tests measuring spatial ability and perceptual speed are shown in Table 7.

TABLE 7

| | Means scores of groups | | |
	Control $N = 18$	Experimental $N = 4$	Significance
Perceptual speed (50 items)	17·75	21·5	N.S.
Spatial ability (30 items)	10·25	14·5	0·02

Although the sample size makes extrapolation difficult, the results are similar to other results of training Africans in three-dimensional perception (McFie, 1961; Dawson, 1967).

Even though the discussion of the possibility of improvement of abilities has been limited to spatial ability, it does appear that there is no reason why most of the abilities should not be improved, even at a later stage in impaired children. What is unclear, is the best method of tackling this improvement process and what limitations on development are imposed by early impairment.

A further important area in which information is required is the changing nature of the contribution of different 'abilities' when learning a particular skilled task and the extent to which procedures for effecting this transition can be developed. Although these problems cannot be discussed here, it may be noted that the approach by Hefferline (1958) and Connolly (1968) appear to be promising.

While approaching the problem of the treatment of motor dysfunction from different theoretical positions there appears to be a common emphasis emerging from a number of sources concerning the importance of such basic abilities. Ayres (1963) for example, in discussing what she terms as five major syndromes of perceptual-motor dysfunction, includes among her conclusions the following hypothesis. The development of central nervous system processes of organising and augmenting tactile impulses in association with meaningful experiences must precede the ability to perform skilled motor tasks. It seems that the continuous flow of tactile sensation, if meaningful, lays down in the brain schemata upon which all future motor planning is based. This aspect is discussed further in relation to the developing 'body image' (page 123).

References

Abercrombie, M. L. (1964) *Perceptual and visuo-motor disorders in cerebral palsy.* London: Heinemann.

Altman, J. & Das, G. D. (1964) A radiographic examination of the effects of an enriched environment in the adult rat brain. *Nature,* 204, 1161–1165.

Ayres, A. J. (1963) The development of perceptual-motor abilities: a theoretical basis for treatment of dysfunction. *Amer. J. Occup. Therapy,* 17, 6, 221–225.

Bagley, W. C. (1900) On the correlation of mental and motor ability in schoolchildren. *Am. J. Psych.,* 12, 193–205.

Bennet, E. L., Diamond, M. C. & Krech, D. & Rosenweig, M. R. (1964) Chemical and anatomical plasticity of the brain. *Science,* 146, 610–619.

Bijou, S. W. & Baer, D. M. (1963) Some methodological contributions from a functional analysis of child development. *Adv. Child Devel. Behav.,* 1, 197–231.

Bobath, K. (1966) *The motor deficit in patients with cerebral palsy.* London: Heinemann.

Brace, D. K. (1932) Why P.E. is a way of education. J. *Health & P.E.,* 3, 20–54.

Brenner, M. W., Gillman, S., Zangwill, O. L. & Farrel, M. (1967) Visuo motor ability in schoolchildren. *Brit. M. J.,* 4, 259–262.

Broadbent, D. E. (1958) *Perception & Communication.* Oxford: Pergamon.

Buhler, C. (1935) From birth to maturity. London: Kegan Paul.

Caldwell, E. M. (1956) A case of spatial inability in a cerebral palsied child. British Council for Welfare of Spastics.

Carmichael, J. (1952) *Manual of child psychology.* New York: Wiley.

Chaney, C. M. & Kephart, M. C. (1968) *Motoric aids to perceptual training.* Ohio: Merrill.

Connolly, K. (1968) The application of operant conditioning to the measurement and development of motor skill in children. *Dev. Med. Child. Neur.*, 106, 697–705.

Corah, N. L. *et al.* (1968) Effects of perinatal anoxia after seven years. *Psych. Monogr.*, 79, 3, 1–33.

Cruickshank, W. M., Bice, A. T. & Waller, B. (1957) *Perception and cerebral palsy*: a study in figure-background relationship. Syracuse: University Press.

Dawson, J. L. M. (1967) Cultural and physiological influences upon spatial perceptual processes in West Africa. *Int. J. Psych.*, 2, 115–122.

Deutsch, J. A. (1960) *The structural basis of behaviour.* Chicago: University Press.

Di Stefano, M. K., Ellis, N. & Sloan, W. (1958) Motor proficiency in mental defectives. *Percept. & Motor Skills*, 8, 231–234.

Dodwell, P. O. (1964) A coupling system for coding and learning in shape discrimination. *Psych. Rev.*, 71, 148–159.

Doll, E. A. (1946) The Oseretzky scale. *Am. J. Ment. Def.*, 50, 485–487.

Doman, G. & Delacato, C. H. (1967) *A summary of concepts, procedures and organisation.* Institute for the Achievement of Human Potential.

Espenchade, A. (1940) Motor performance in adolescence. *Monog. Soc. Res. Child Dev.*, 5.

Fairweather, O. V. & Illsley, R. (1960) Obstetric and social origins of mentally handicapped children. *Brit. J. Prev. Soc. Med.*, 14, 149–159.

Fantz, R. L. (1967) Visual perception and experience in early infancy. In H. W. Stevenson, E. H. Hess & H. L. Rheingold (Eds.) *Early behaviour, comparative and developmental approaches.* New York: Wiley.

Farmer, E. (1927) A group factor in sensory motor tests. *Brit. J. Psych.*, 17, 4, 327–342.

Fish, B. (1961) The study of motor development in infancy and its relation to psychological functioning. *Am. J. Psychiat.*, 17, 113–118.

Fleishman, E. A. (1954) Dimensional analysis of psychomotor abilities. *J. Exp. Psych.*, 48, 437–454.

Fleishman, E. A. (1967) Individual differences and motor learning. In R. M. Gagne (Ed.) *Individual differences.* Ohio: Merrill.

French, J. W. (1951) The description of aptitudes and achievement tests in terms of rotated factors. *Psychometric Mono.*, 5.

Garfield, E. (1923) The measurement of motor ability. *Arch. Psych.*, 62.

Garfield, J. C. (1964) Motor impersistence in normal and brain-damaged children. *Neurology*, 14, 623–630.

Garfield, J. C., Benton, A. L. & McQueen, J. C. (1966) Motor impersistence in brain-damaged and cultural-familial defectives. *J. Nerv. Ment. Dis.*, 42, 434–440.

Gesell, A. (1928) *Infancy and human growth.* New York: Macmillan.

Gibson, E. J. (1953)   Improvement in perceptual judgements as a function of controlled practice of training. *Psych. Bull.*, 50, 6, 401–431.

Gibson, E. J. & Gibson, J. J. (1962)   Developmental study of the discrimination of letter-like forms. *J. Comp. Physiol. Psych.*, 55, 897–906.

Gibson, H. B. (1964)   The spiral maze. A psychomotor test with implications for the study of delinquency. *Brit. J. Psych.*, 54, 219–225.

Gibson, H. B. (1965)   *Manual of the Gibson Spiral Maze.* London: University Press.

Graham, F. K. & Kendall, B. S. (1960)   *Memory for designs test.* Revised general manual. *Percept. Motor Skills*, 11, 147–188.

Greenberg, D. A., Uzgiris, I. C. & Hunt, J. McV (1968)   The effect of visual stimulation upon the blink response of human infants. *J. Genetic Psych.*, 113, 167–176.

Griffiths, R. (1954)   *The abilities of babies.* London: University Press.

Hebb, D. O. (1939)   The intelligence in man after the removal of cerebral tissue. *J. Genet. Psych.*, 21, 73–87.

Hebb, D. O. (1949)   *The organization of behaviour.* New York: Wiley.

Hefferline, R. F. (1958)   The role of proprioception in the control of behaviour. *Trans. New York Ac., Sci.*, 20, 739.

Hershenson, M. Musinger, H. & Hessen, W. (1965)   Preferences for shapes of intermediate variability in the newborn human. *Science*, 144, 315–317.

Hershenson, M. (1967)   Development of perception of form. *Psych. Bull.*, 326–336.

Hurlock, E. B. (1949)   *Child growth and development.* New York: McGraw-Hill.

Illingworth, R. (1963)   *Development of the infant and young child.* London: Livingstone.

Ismail, A. H. & Gruber, J. J. (1967)   *Motor aptitude and intellectual performance.* Ohio: Merrill.

Johnson, G. B. (1932)   Physical skill test for sectioning classes into homogeneous groups. *Res. Quart.*, 3, 128–138.

Kephart, N. C. (1960)   *The slow learner in the classroom.* Ohio: Merrill.

Kessen, N., Haith, M. M. & Salapatek, P. (1965)   The ocular orientations of newborn infants to visual contours. Referred to in R. N. Haber (Ed.) (1968) *Contemporary theory and research in visual perception.* New York: Holt, Rinehart & Winston.

Lieberman, R. (1962)   Retinal cholinesterase and glycolysis in rats raised in darkness. *Science*, 135, 372–373.

Lipsitt, L. P. (1969)   Learning capacities of the human infant. In R. J. Robinson (Ed.) *Brain and early behaviour.* London: Academic Press.

McCloy, C. H. (1934)   The measurement of general motor capacities and general motor ability. *Res. Quart.*, 5, 49.

McFie, J. (1961)   The effect of education on African performance on a group of intellectual tasks. *Brit. J. Educ. Psych.*, 31, 232–240.

Malpass, L. F. (1959)   Responses of retarded and normal children to *selected clinical measures*. South Illinois: University Press.

Malpass, L. F. (1960)   Motor proficiency in institutionalised and non-institutionalised retarded and normal children. *Am. J. Ment. Def.*, 64, 1012–1015.

Malpass, L. F. (1963)   Motor skills in mental deficiency. In N. R. Ellis (Ed.) *Handbook of mental deficiency*. New York: McGraw-Hill.

Morgan, C. T. & King, R. A. (1966)   *Introduction to psychology*. New York: McGraw-Hill.

Michael, W. B., Guilford, J. P. Fruchter, B., & Zimmerman, W. S. (1957)   The description of spatial visualisation abilities. *Educ. Psych. Measure.*, 17, 185–199.

Norman, D. A. (1968)   Toward a theory of memory and attention. *Psych. Rev.*, 75, 522–536.

Piaget, J. (1952)   *The origins of intelligence in children*. New York: International Universities Press.

Piaget, J. (1953)   *The origins of intelligence in the child*. London: Routledge & Kegan Paul.

Poole, H. (1969)   Restructuring the perceptual world of African children. *Teacher Education in New Countries*, 10, 2, 165–172.

Porteus, S. D. (1959)   *The maze test and clinical psychology*. California: Pacific Books.

Rabin, H. M. (1957)   The relationships of age, intelligence and sex to motor proficiency in mental defectives. *Am. J. Ment. Def.*, 62, 507–516.

Radin, N. & Sonquist, H. (1968)   Ypsilanti public schools Gale preschool program. Mimeographed final report (from the authors).

Ray, H. C. (1940)   Inter-relationships of mental and physical abilities and achievement of highschool boys. *Res. Quart.*, 11, 129–141.

Reitan, R. M. (1958)   Validity of the trail making test as an indicator of organic brain damage. *Percept. & Motor Skills*, 8, 271–276.

Sackett, G. P. A. (1963)   A neural mechanism underlying unlearned critical periods and developmental aspects of visually controlled behaviour. *Psych. Rev.*, 70, 40–50.

Salapatek, P. & Kessen, N. (1966)   Visual scanning of triangles by the human newborn. *J. Exp. Child. Psych.*, 3, 155–167.

Sapir, G. S. & Wilson, B. M. (1967)   Patterns of developmental deficits. *Percept. & Motor Skills*, 24, 1291–1293.

Seashore, R. H., Buxton, C. E. & McCollan, I. N. (1940)   Multiple factorial analysis of fine motor skills. *Amer. J. Psych.*, 53, 251–259.

Siskind, G. (1966)   Selected designs. A screening device for the children of cerebral dysfunction. *Percept. & Motor Skills*, 23, 811–813.

Sloan, W. (1948)   *Lincoln adaptation of the Oseretzky Scale*. Illinois: Lincoln.

Sloan, W. (1955) The Lincoln–Oseretzky motor developmental scale. *Genetic Psych. Monog.*, 51, 182–252.

Smith, I. M. (1954) The development of a spatial test. *Durham Res. Rev.*, 5, 19–33.

Smith, I. M. (1964) *Spatial abilities*. London: University Press.

Stechler, G. (1964) The effect of medication during labour on newborn attention. *Science*, 144, 315–317.

Stott, D. H. (1966) A general test of motor-impairment for children. *Dev. Med. Child. Neur.*, 8, 523–531.

Strauss, A. A. & Kephart, N. C. (1955) *Psychopathology and education of the brain-injured child*. New York: Grave & Stratton.

Sutherland, N. (1959) Stimulus analysing mechanisms. In *Mechanisation of thought processes*. London: H.M.S.O.

Tamburrini, J. (1968) Piaget in perspective. Paper presented at a conference in the School of Education—University of Sussex.

Thurstone, I. L. (1950) *A factorial study of perception*. Chicago: University Press.

Treisman, A. M. (1969) Strategies and models of selective attention. *Psych. Rev.*, 76, 3, 282–299.

Vernon, P. E. (1950) *The structure of human abilities*, London: Methuen.

Vernon, M. (1957) *Backwardness in reading*. New York: Cambridge University Press.

Walk, R. D. & Gibson, E. J. (1961) A comparative analytical study of depth perception. *Psych. Monog.*, 75, 15.

Wechsler, D. (1949) *W.I.S.C.* New York: Psychological Corporation.

Weiskrantz, L. (1958) Sensory deprivation and the cat's optic nerve system. *Nature*, 181, 1047–1050.

Welton, J. (1912) *The psychology of education*, London: Macmillan.

White, B. L. (1969) The initial coordination of sensori-motor schemas in human infants. In D. Elkind & J. A. Flavell (Eds.) *Studies in Cognitive Development*. New York: Oxford University Press.

White, B. L. & Held, R. (1966) Plasticity of sensori-motor development in the human infant. In J. F. Rosenblith & W. Alinsmith (Eds.) *The courses of behaviour*. New York: Allyn & Bacon.

Whiting, H. T. A., Johnson, G. F. & Page, M. (1969a) The Gibson Spiral Maze as a possible screening device for minimal brain damage. *Brit. J. Soc. Clin. Psych.*, 8, 164–168.

Whiting, H. T. A., Johnson, G. F. & Page, M. (1969b) Factor analytic study of motor impairment at the ten-year age level in normal and E.S.N. populations. Unpublished paper, Physical Education Dept., Leeds University.

Whiting, H. T. A., Davies, J. G., Gibson, J. M., Lumley, R., Sutcliffe, R. S. E. & Morris, P. R. (1970) Motor impairment in an approved school population. Unpublished paper, Physical Education Department, Leeds University.

Wisler, C. (1901) The correlation of mental and physical tests. *Psych. Rev. Monog. Supp.*

Witkin, H. A., Dyk, R. B., Faterson, M. F. & Karp, S. A. (1962) *Psychological differentiation.* New York: Wiley.

Wober, M. (1965) Sensotypes. *J. Soc. Psych.*, 70, 181–189.

Yarmolenko, A. (1933) The motor sphere of school children. *J. Genet Psych.*, 42, 298–316.

Yates, P. T. (1968) Abnormalities of psychomotor function. In H. J. Eysenck (Ed.) *Handbook of abnormal psychology*, London: Pergamon.

CHAPTER 4

Motor Impairment and the Socialisation Process

> *The human infant enters this world at some place on its*
> *surface and finds himself among adults who have certain*
> *stable ways of behaving towards physical objects and in*
> *social situations and who use a language which has a cer-*
> *tain codification. Gradually, he learns to behave like*
> *others do, i.e. learns the culture and in so doing simultan-*
> *eously develops elaborate systems of cognitions (ways of*
> *perceiving, meanings, associations, attitudes and so*
> *forth) and also simultaneously he learns the language,*
> *associating auditory stimulus patterns with cognitions*
> *(decoding) and cognitions with verbal behaviour (encoding)*
> *both according to the rules of the code. Given this complete*
> *interweaving of culture, cognition and language in the*
> *course of development, it is not surprising that social*
> *scientists later find it difficult to disentangle the threads.*
> *The greatest single pitfall in the way of research in this*
> *area is thus circularity of inferences.*
>
> (Osgood & Sebeck, 1954)

The socialisation process as Osgood & Sebeck elaborate is a
complex one and if it is difficult to tease out effects which are
responsible for specific behaviour patterns, it is perhaps even
more difficult to attribute deviant behaviour to particular
influences or their absence. Such patterns must be viewed
within their historical context. As Dunsdon (1952) has pointed
out:

> The importance of obtaining developmental histories as
> detailed as possible will be obvious, since the degree to which
> a child was making use of his abilities needed to be assessed
> in the light of such matters as the age at which he was first
> able to sit, walk and speak, or to communicate his needs

by other means and the effect of any concomitant sensory disabilities on his efforts towards independence.

Unfortunately, developmental histories are usually obtained in retrospect and the difficulties involved and the relative unreliability of the information are familiar to any worker in this field.

Learning to communicate and to acquire the complex social patterns of the group is the result of a socialisation process which initiates with the parents and is continued and fostered by the peer group and the community at large. Stevenson (1965) considers adult approval is the most commonly used means of affecting behaviour. Adult approval of social behaviour is known as a social reinforcer. Baer *et al.* (1963) showed that as the child grows older he depends less and less on social reinforcers to guide his behaviour and is more likely to use direct information from the situation as a lead to his responses. Buhler (1933) summarised three stages of socialisation resulting in three types of social behaviour:

1. Socially blind
2. Socially dependent
3. Socially independent

Social blindness is the state apparently before the baby is aware of the social pressures and events around him. His social behaviour is limited to his need for attention and survival. Socially dependent behaviour arises when actions are socially reinforced by the adult parental figure and social behaviour arises only within the structure of parental or adult security.

Possible links between behaviour disorders and motor impairment were suggested in Chapter 2 particularly in relation to known instances of brain damage. The study reported by Knobloch & Pasamanick (1959) for example showed a connection between motor deficits, behaviour disorders in childhood and brain damage. Again, Pasamanick *et al.* (1956) and Rogers *et al.* (1955) showed positive significant correlations between behaviour disturbances at school and certain complications of pregnancy. In a follow-up study after an interval of 7 years on a known group who had experienced prenatal anoxia, postnatal apnea or both, Corah *et al.* (1965) reported impairment in perceptual skill and *social competence*. The oft-quoted idea of a brain-injured personality indexed by a syndrome consisting of traits such as hyperactivity, impulsivity, distractibility, irritability and emotional lability (Strauss & Kephart, 1955; Clements & Peters, 1962; Silver, 1958) was not supported in this study. This is in keeping with Eisenberg's (1964) suggestion that:

> the greatest fallacy of all is the common assumption that there is *a* brain damage syndrome.

In the Corah *et al.* study only impulsivity and distractibility were significantly different in the anoxic group as compared with a control group. The anoxics further achieved a significantly lower mean score on the Vineland Social Quotient Scale.

A further general finding was that the anoxics tended to show more dependent behaviour than normals.* A significantly greater number of the postnatal subgroup of anoxics and the subgroup with a guarded prognosis showed deficits in motor coordination as assessed by teacher's ratings.

At a more subjective level, parents of 'clumsy' children as already quoted (page 37) also stress the social implications of impairment:

> suffers socially with children who are aware of his handicap.

> . . . perhaps it is too late psychologically to help my child because the scars of ridicule by other children and his own awareness of his lack of ability and my own over-protectiveness might be too deep.

> He has lost two of his neighbourhood buddies because he can't play ball well enough to suit them and that is all they want to do. The fact that he does better than they in school doesn't seem to console him when he wants to play.

Possible interpretations of why a linkage between motor impairment and socialisation should be manifest, is the subject matter of parts of this chapter. Three main issues would seem to be worth elaborating:

1. In relation to the model of perceptual-motor skill performance established in Chapter 1 (which it will be recalled

---

*An interesting side issue in relation to dependent behaviour is Radin & Sonquist's (1968) finding that children who enter pre-school with habits of dependency are more open to influence, and hence to cognitive stimulation by teaching staff thus reinforcing desirable responses. Walters & Parke (1964) suggest that the way in which dependency facilitates learning is by the development of habits of orienting and attending to adults.

applies equally well to the acquisition of social skills) *selective attention/perception* was shown to be essential to the efficient learning of skills. In this respect, it is of interest to note Richardson's (1964) reminder that the brain-damaged child has difficulty in focusing his attention selectively and sustaining it:

> In the extreme he is at the mercy of every extraneous sight and sound in his environment. He fails to apprehend what is of moment because he is distracted by the trivial and the transient.

2. Rogers *et al.* (1955) have raised the interesting consideration that since behaviour problems in children are very often attributed to the tension in their mother, serious consideration should be given to the other side of the picture, i.e. whether or not the infant with difficulties first produced the tension.

3. The 'status significance' that competence in physical skills carries at particular stages of childhood and the effect this might have on development of the individual's 'self-esteem'. Such activities as riding a bicycle, skipping, skating, walking on stilts or tin cans and catching a ball particularly come to mind. These are reasonably high grade skills but which the majority of children given a reasonable practice period manage to acquire.

These three sections will now be developed in some detail.

Selective attention/perception

This topic has already been raised a number of times particularly in relation to the general skill model and the development of spatial ability. It is not surprising to find it listed again under the general heading of the socialisation process because as Argyle & Kendon (1967) suggest:

> It is fruitful to look upon the behaviour of people engaged in focused interaction as an organised, skilled performance analogous to car-driving.

A failure to acquire social skills will inhibit social interaction and vice versa.

In relation to the development of spatial ability (page 88) it was pointed out how infants have certain innate patterns of perceptual response. Fantz's (1967) work in particular suggests that the very young infant can selectively respond to spatial configurations of the human face. Social skills depend upon developed abilities amongst which selective perception figures prominently. For example, variations in sound—such as the different tones of the human voice—are being assimilated and practised by the infant some time before words are used for the purposes of communication. Similarly, the control of the musculature is necessary before appropriate gestures, facial and bodily, are used in social interaction.

The process of socialisation has been described by Bell (1962) as:

> . . . the process by which the child, whose behaviour and personality are undifferentiated, is moulded into an adult that is acceptable to the society in which he lives.

These definitions are typical of the general view which is taken of socialisation. They imply an interaction between the mother or mother-substitute which extends to other members of the family, peers and ultimately society at large. What is often missed in these definitions is comment about the 'equipment' the child needs to possess to gain from social interaction. Hardman (1970) suggests that *accurate perceptual mechanisms* constitute such 'equipment'. He proposes that the basis for perceptual development while being partly innately determined is laid down in the early months during a process which he terms *primary socialisation* and on this depends future social learning which might be designated *secondary socialisation*.

The extent to which primary socialisation is effective depends on the nature of the affective relationship between the mother and the child in that the quality of such a relationship will influence the quantity and quality of sensory stimulation the mother makes available to the child.

> Social behaviour is behaviour that is evoked, maintained and modified by the presence or behaviour of another organism usually by a member of one's own species. Social stimuli, those provided by these organisms, differ from inanimate stimuli in more than origin, they are often more responsive and more unpredictable, more variable, more flexible and more likely to be intermittent.
>
> (Skinner, 1953)

The tenor of the present discussion is that primary socialisation represents the establishment of information processing abilities related to the kinds of display involved in social interaction. A failure or limitation in such primary socialisation will result in a failure or delay in social interaction and social competence. Thus, the objective of primary socialisation is to give adequate sensory experiences of a diverse kind and particularly within a social framework. In as far as the newborn needs to differentiate between himself and others, touch and pressure stimuli will play an important part in relation to early development of the concept of 'I' (Chapter 5).

It would seem apparent that in order for such stimulation possibility to be maximally effective, the emotional bond between parent and child should be satisfactory. Estrangement could result in reduction in social interaction between the two; particularly of the playful type of behaviour often indulged in by parents. Such reduction would indirectly result in reduced experience and hence sensory perceptual deprivation. That such deprivation is disadvantageous to the human infant is borne out by studies on hospitalised or institutionalised children such as those reported earlier (pages 62–63) by Schaffer (1965, 1966) and Schaffer & Emerson (1968).

In addition, Durfee & Wolf as long ago as 1933 suggested two broad classifications of reasons underlying the psychological insult suffered by institutionalised children:

1. Lack of stimulation. In many cases, the worst offenders would appear to be the best equipped and most hygienic institutions, which succeed in sterilising the surroundings of the child from germs but which at the same time sterilise the child's psyche. Even bad parents, the most destitute of homes and poor environmental conditions offer more mental stimulation than the usual hospital ward.

2. The presence or absence of the child's mother. Stimulation by the mother will always be more intensive than that of even the best trained nursery personnel, though the replacement of the natural mother by a mother-substitute has good results especially if at adoption the age of the child is below seven months.

While paediatricians for many years have suspected that the cause of hospitalism was related in some vague way to the infant's psyche experimental results have not been forthcoming and might still be looked upon as suggestive rather than conclusive. Czerny (1922) for example concluded that hospitalism was due to lack of adequate stimulation and felt that monotony together with staring at blank walls and ceilings were important factors. Kaupe (1920) emphasised the role of the mother:

> The psychic and physical influence of the mother was a very important weapon against hospitalism.

Brenneman (1932) recognised the effects of the absence of mothering and had a rule in his hospital that every baby should be picked up, carried around, amused and 'mothered' several times a day. Talbot (1941) recounting an experience he had in 1900 during a visit to a children's clinic in Dusseldorf. He noticed a very fat old lady wandering about the ward with a very measly baby on her hip. He asked Schlossman, the Director, who she was and he was told that whenever they had a baby for whom they had done everything medically possible and were unsuccessful, they turned the baby over to old Anna and told her to take charge. Old Anna was always successful. No doubt this is rather an emotionally charged story but it is an example of 'instinctive' care that subsequent research has supported.

Tension in the mother

The presence of a mother or mother substitute who interacts with the child providing care, stimulation and an emotional bond would on the above evidence appear to be essential for adequate development. However, such a relationship is not a one-way relationship—it is an interaction process. The child who is impaired in motor skill performance or deficient in certain socially desired skills (such as the ability to walk at roughly the expected time within a given culture) might prove a source of embarrassment to his parents resulting in tension and his being deprived of experience in many situations in which his social behaviour might have the opportunity to develop. As Barker & Wright (1955) suggest, such children will have a more restricted social environment. Richardson (1964) extrapolating from the work of Fairweather & Illsley (1960) suggests that a child may exhibit forms of malfunctioning often associated with brain injury even though the aetiological factors derive almost wholly from his lack of some of the experiences necessary for adequate socialisation. The point being made here, is that such children are not only limited by their own disabilities *per se*, but also by the reactions of themselves and others to such disabilities. The reaction of the child to his own disabilities is perhaps a more obvious one and will be further reinforced when he enters the play situation with other children:

> They laugh at me, and I turn away
> Look at them!
> Dear God why do I have to live?
> Why did it happen to me?
> They laugh and call me names;
> Wicked, evil, upsetting names.
> My mother tries to comfort me,
> But I know I will never be like them.
>
> I sit, staring at the playing field,
> The boys play happily.
> I wish, oh I wish that
> I could run about like others.
> All I can do is watch
> From my spastic's chair
>
> (Poem by Neil Best—age 13)

The effect that a child suffering from motor impairment may have on others with whom he may come into contact is not well documented. In this respect, Richardson (1964) has commented:

> This fragmentary evidence suggests that certain malfunctions in children may so disturb the persons responsible for his socialisation as to further jeopardise a child's chance of obtaining the varieties of experience he needs for adequate socialisation. Additional work is needed to examine the extent to which different syndromes of malfunctioning have disturbing effects on other people and whether the degree and type of disturbance varies with different cultural and sub-cultural contents.

Inadequate emotional response on the part of the mother could result from her own personality, i.e. the cold, aloof, cycloid type would, presumably, find the warm maternal response more difficult. Again, such factors as post-puerperal depression lasting, in some cases, for nine months, could disturb normal emotional behaviour on the part of the mother. The personality and temperament of the baby will influence the mother's reaction. The use of phrases, such as 'a good baby' or 'a difficult baby' reflect the subjective assessments which are continually made. Casler (1968) acknowledges the influence of the baby's personality:

> It seems safe to say that the less attractive and responsive the baby is the less positive will be the mother's attitudes towards it.

The term 'less positive' would suggest a possible reduction in the handling of, and playing with the baby. It could well be that the minimally brain-damaged child might be in 'the difficult baby' category. Prechtl (1963) in a study of 1,000 babies during the first nine days of life, identified a set of distinct syndromes of minimal brain damage and showed that the mothers did not know of this and that:

> . . . the behaviour patterns (i.e. of the babies) were a source of distress, worry, and grief to the mother.

In a longitudinal study of some of these brain-damaged children Prechtl noticed that in seven out of eight of the abnormal babies the mothers did not show a harmonious positive attitude to the baby after a few months. This attitude was noticed in only *one* mother in a 'control' group of ten babies. Prechtl concluded that:

> Abnormal behaviour in an infant can influence and change the mothering and maternal attitude. Neurologically abnormal babies do not make adequate partners in the child-mother interaction.

Further evidence for this reaction occurring comes from the data on impaired children which shows a link with prematurity. This in itself can be disadvantageous as the 'prematurity synodrome', described by Montague (1950), is seen as high emotion, proneness to naso-pharangeal and respiratory infections and behaviour disorders, e.g. in feeding.

Such a combination of factors which tend to lessen the baby's attractiveness, prompted Stott (1962) to say:

> Children who failed to pass the adoption or mothering test on account of one observed congenital impairment would be more likely to exhibit others, some of which . . . would only be apparent later.

It is interesting to note that this argument for a link between minimal brain damage and rejection or partial rejection of the child is not disproved by the findings of Hewett *et al.* (1970). They find that parents of severely handicapped children 'claim' to have no feelings of revulsion. However, one wonders to what extent the diagnosis of 'handicapped' puts the child, and his parents, in a situation where sympathy is shown and allowances made. It is feasible that such allowances are not made where the dysfunction is minimal and seen purely as clumsiness or awkwardness and where, because of the absence of clinical diagnosis, the child is expected to be normal.

Status significant motor skills

Evidence of the social acceptability of children was shown by Northway (1966) to develop as early as four years of age. In a study of thirty-six pre-school children of 4 years, the children showed clear differentiation of social acceptability to one another, and considerable consistency of acceptability for different activities. It was felt, that with the least and most acceptable children, the level of maturity may correspond to acceptability. Differences in a few months at this age may correspond to quite a marked degree in social skills, and these skills count for acceptability. Northway (1966) speculated that precocity of social skills, in nursery age children, related to a higher degree of sensori-motor skill development. She suggested that the child who was slower at developing sensori-motor skills was held back—he was still struggling to fasten buttons, or cut out a paper pattern, when the precocious child was already on to the next pursuit—interacting with his teacher or other children, helping others, being sent on messages; all experiences which were widening his social horizon.

Hewett *et al.* (1970) quote a parent:

> At the table for example the child with poor hand control might often drop cups and spill food, for which in fairness he could not be chastised, although his brothers and sisters might be.

In this case the mother had to try to explain to the other children of the justice of her decision and, whatever the outcome, the status of the 'clumsy' child is reduced. Furthermore, only the most naïve could believe that this attitude is not conveyed to the child, thus affecting his self-concept.

An essential point to note from the evidence is that the 'clumsy' child is in a particularly disadvantageous state— more so than the clinically diagnosed child. Hewett *et al.* (1970) make this point:

> The two groups of children who seemed to have most difficulty fitting into the ordinary play situation with normal children were those whose physical handicaps were just severe enough to make it impossible to keep up with the others in all their activities, but not severe enough for the other children to make allowances for them, and the mentally handicapped.

With older children, Sutton-Smith & Roberts (1964) extrapolating from the 'games-theory' classification of games:

1. games of chance
2. games of physical skill
3. games of strategy

proposes three categories of competitor:

1. fortunists who rely on luck to succeed
2. potents who achieve success by physical skill
3. strategists who succeed by wise decision

They were able to show in one study (Sutton-Smith & Roberts, 1964) that 50% of boys and girls named by teachers as successful in the playground were in the top quarter of the distribution of 'potents' rankings. Thirty-four potents as against seventeen strategists were classified by the teacher as playground successes.

A similar finding was reported by Jones & Bayley (1950) in their attempt to find differentiating behavioural characteristics between two extreme groups of boys. Two groups of boys who were opposite in status on the basis of one developmental characteristic (skeletal age) were selected. Social behaviour was determined by the Institute of Child Welfare ratings. Descriptive data on each boy was obtained. Ratings and observations were made in mixed group situations. Reputation tests obtained from classmates were recorded. It was found that those who are physically accelerated are usually accepted and treated by adults and other children as more mature. Early maturing boys appear to have relatively little need to strive for status. The physically retarded boys exhibit many forms of immature behaviour.

Motor impairment and maladjustment

Although evidence from studies already quoted (Lilienfeld *et al.*, 1955, Rogers *et al.*, 1955, Corah *et al.*, 1965) does indicate that minimal brain damage may result in perceptual-motor impairment and social incompetence, it would be wrong (as emphasised in the previous chapters) to assume that all cases of such impairment reflect brain damage. Whiting *et al.* (1970) for example in a study on an approved school population between the ages of 11.0 years and 14.0 years were able to show that sixteen of the sample of sixty boys were suffering from motor impairment (on the criterion adopted). In only four cases was there some firm evidence of brain damage (two of these involved fractured skulls during childhood). The majority of the evidence seemed to favour environmental causation. The average birthweight of the impaired group was 5 lb. $15\frac{1}{2}$ oz. and the number of children in each family averaged 5·7 (range 2–10). From the records (which may have been inadequate), only one premature birth was reported and four cases involved pregnancy complications. In addition, the following adverse environmental conditions (rarely encountered singly) were noted:

> Delinquent sub-culture, criminal parents, impoverished home environment, separation, divorce, co-habitation, step-parents, maternal or paternal deprivation, psychotic parent, physically handicapped parent, violence in the home, cruelty, rejection, institutionalisation, illegitimacy, over-indulgence, under-nourishment and emotional deprivation.

A reinforcement to the words of Osgood & Sebeck with which this chapter opened.

Stott (1959, 1962, 1964) perhaps more than any other worker has linked 'motor impairment' with maladjustment and delinquency. He hypothesised a factor of congenital impairment. By congenital Stott (1959) implies that the antecedents of the condition date from birth or before (i.e. including factors operating during gestation or delivery).

Stott's syndrome of somatic or neural impairment is a loose one, containing a number of alternative manifestations any one of which appears in only a minority of the cases. Thus, behaviour disturbance as a component of the syndrome could be the sole symptom. Although on the basis of the skill model previously proposed, this would seldom appear to be the case.

Stott (1962) suggests that *if* the behaviour disturbance is seen as part of a syndrome of:

1. Pregnancy
2. Multiple impairment, e.g. mental subnormality
   susceptibility to common infections
   delayed growth
   congenital malformation
3. Brain damage, e.g. epilepsy
   motor impairment
   strabismus
   speech defect
   organic dysfunction
   failure of homeostasis

then its organic origin is more likely. This would be supported by the work of Lilienfeld *et al.*, Rogers *et al.* and Corah *et al.* previously discussed. In this paper, Stott did in fact present general epidemiological evidence for a congenital factor in the behaviour disturbance of boys nearly all of whom would be within a normal range of intelligence and attending state schools.

A deduction made by Stott on the basis of his syndrome of pregnancy-multiple impairment was that disturbed delinquents would be more likely than the stable to suffer physical ill-health, defect or abnormalities of growth. In a study of Glasgow probationers (Stott, 1962) he was able to show that the more disturbed among the probationers and a non-delinquent control group were more prone to chronic disease and physical defects. He suggests the possibility of 'constitutional' damage to the child's temperament.

Stott further compared the incidence of five categories of physical defect, ill-health and abnormality of growth found within the different degrees of behaviour disturbance as recorded by his Bristol Social Adjustment Guide scores. The maladjusted (20 or more points on the B.S.A.G.) were between $3\frac{1}{2}$ times and $4\frac{1}{2}$ times more liable to chronic ill-health than the temperamentally stable children (0–4 points); 4 times more liable to have physical defects; nearly 3 times as liable to have bad eyesight and over 3 times more likely to be of abnormal growth (diminutive, very fat, very thin, etc.).

In a further study of thirty-three troublesome children (Stott, 1964) he found that the salient feature among a group of five of them from stable families was somatic or neural impairment. Two of the children were enuretic, one epileptic, two had speech defects and two had unnatural body posture. In three out of the five cases, the mothers reported some complication during pregnancy or birth. Considering the group as a whole, there was a high incidence of somatic or neural impairment affecting twenty-six of the thirty-three cases. Where there were symptoms indicating neural damage (of congenital origin) there was a significant excess of other somatic or neural impairment.

On the basis of this work, Stott was forced to consider the possibility that behaviour disturbances were part of a syndrome which has its origins in some type of congenital or neural impairment which is aggravated when the affected person is exposed to a stressful situation.

While some support for the pregnancy multiple impairment hypothesis in relation to delinquency comes from the previously cited paper (Whiting *et al.*, 1970) where amongst the case histories of some of the motor-impaired group were reported symptoms of neural somatic dysfunction (including speech, hearing and sight defects), enuresis, deformity, serious illness and anxiety and stress during pregnancy, the incidence of such cases was low.

Further support for Stott's findings, however, comes from Drillien (1964) and Prechtl (1961) who report that complications during pregnancy and delivery are strongly associated with behaviour disturbance at a later stage. Drillien's evidence also confirms the hypothesis that familial stress brings congenital impairment to the surface.

In his longitudinal study on the growth and development of prematurely born infants, Drillien (1964) suggested that:

> . . . behaviour disturbance in school was found to be increased when there was a history of severe complications of pregnancy and/or delivery and also when the child had suffered severe familial stress in the pre-school period.

Bamber (1966) provides more recent support for some of Stott's contentions. In a study of an approved school population, he found that 35% of the sample had histories of complications during pregnancy or at delivery. Evidence was also produced in support of Stott's theory of multiple congenital defects. He suggested that approved school children were more likely to show symptoms of brain damage or neural impairment (not supported in the Whiting *et al.*, 1970 study). Postnatal environmental stress such as illegitimacy, death of mother/father, desertion by one parent, divorce, unemployment of father, physical neglect, etc., were still the most common factors in the histories of his approved school group.

Brain damage, personality and socialisation

An interesting linkage can be made between personality theory in Eysenck's (1968a) terms, brain damage and the socialisation process.

Briefly, Eysenck has proposed (and provided limited evidence for over a number of years) the existence of two orthogonal dimensions (continuua) of personality designated extraversion/introversion and neuroticism (stable/unstable). More recently (Eysenck, 1968b; Eysenck & Eysenck, 1969) a third major orthogonal dimension of psychoticism has received extended treatment and it seems likely that developments in this area will follow.

The dimension of extraversion/introversion is related to the rate of build-up of reactive inhibition in the cortex and the generation of cortical excitation. The more extraverted person generates reactive inhibition relatively quickly and excitation relatively slowly. The reverse state applies for a person more towards the introverted end of the continuum. The implication of such a proposition is that the more introverted person will form conditioned reflexes relatively quickly and strongly while the more extraverted person under similar conditioning situations will acquire conditioned reflexes relatively slowly and such reflexes will be relatively weakly established. Moreover, once conditioned responses are formed in the introverted person, the more difficult they will be to extinguish when compared with such responses in the more extraverted person.

In terms of socialisation, it is proposed by Eysenck that individuals within a particular culture undergo similar socialisation procedures which in the early years in particular are mediated to a large extent by conditioning. Thus, within particular cultures, the introverted person will tend to be over-socialised while the extraverted person will tend to be under-socialised.

Blakemore (1968) following on Eysenck, has accumulated evidence to the effect that groups of brain-damaged subjects are slow to acquire conditioned responses when compared with control subjects but this does not necessarily apply to *all* brain-damaged subjects. The onset of brain-damage would appear to be at least one of the ways in which 'personality change' might be mediated. Blakemore discusses such change as follows:

> In terms of Eysenck's theory it would follow that injury of the brain would interfere with the reciprocal exchange of neural impulses between the cortex and the reticular activating system thus increasing the effects of suppressor mechanisms. The results of brain damage would therefore be related to increased cortical inhibition, leading behaviourally to such effects as slow formation of conditioned responses, swift accumulation of reactive inhibition and extraversion. Evidence in favour of such an hypothesis does exist but it is by no means extensive.

Anderson & Hanvik (1950) have produced evidence for differential effects on personality change dependent upon the site of particular brain lesions. Thus, it would appear (Blakemore's interpretation) that the frontal lobe cases would move towards the extraverted end of the continuum and the parietal lobe cases towards the introverted end resulting in differential effects on aspects of behaviour such as conditioning, learning (including social learning) and perception.

Evidence from impaired populations of a kind with which this book is concerned would not appear to be available at the present time. With cases of minimal impairment there is also the difficulty of diagnosing brain damage and perhaps even greater difficulty in localising such damage. Whiting *et al.* (1970) looked at personality differences between an impaired group (using Stott's test and criteria) and a non-impaired group of 12–14-year-old approved school boys. There were no significant differences between the groups in terms of the personality dimensions of neuroticism and extraversion. The approved school population as a whole were, however, more neurotic than a randomly selected population of school children of similar age. In view of the apparently small number of boys with evidence of brain damage in the group, the failure to find differences which might be attributable to brain damage is understandable.

References

Argyle, M. & Kendon, A. (1967) Experimental analysis of social performance. In L. Berkowitz (Ed.) *Advances in experimental social psychology*, Vol. III, New York: Academic Press.

Anderson, A. L. & Hanvik, L. J. (1950) The psychometric localisation of brain lesions: the differential effect of frontal and parietal lesions on M.M.P.I. profiles. *J. Clin., Psych.*, 6, 177–180.

Baer, D. M., Harris, F. R. & Wolf, M. M. (1963) Control of nursery school children's behaviour by programming social reinforcers from their teachers. Unpublished manuscript, University of Washington.

Bamber, J. (1966) Motor impairment. Unpublished M.A. thesis, University of Glasgow.

Barker, R. G. & Wright, H. F. (1955) *Midwest and its children: the psychological ecology of an American town*. New York: Row & Peterson.

Bell, R. P. (1962) *The sociology of education*. New York: Dorsey.

Blakemore, C. B. (1968) Personality and brain damage. In H. J. Eysenck (Ed.) *The biological basis of personality*. Springfield; Thomas.

Brenneman, J. (1932) The infant ward. *Am. J. Dis. Child*, 43, 577.

Buhler, K. (1933) *The mental development of the child*. London: Routledge & Kegan Paul.

Casler, L. (1968) Perceptual deprivation in institutional settings. In G. Newton & S. Levine (Eds.) *Early experience and behaviour*. Springfield: Thomas.

Clements, S. D. & Peters, J. E. (1962) Minimal brain dysfunction in the school-age child. *Arch. Gen. Psychiat.*, 6, 185–197.

Corah, N. L., Anthony, E. J., Panter, P., Stern, J. A. & Thurston, D. L. (1965) Effects of perinatal anoxia after seven years. *Psych. Monog.*, 79, 3, 1–33.

Czerny, A. (1922) *Der artzt als erzieher des kinder, ed. 6.* Leipzig. Franz Deuticke.

Drillien, C. N. (1964) *Growth and development of prematurely born infants*. Edinburgh: Livingstone.

Dunsdon, M. I. (1952) *The educability of cerebral-palsied children.* London: Newnes.

Durfee, H. & Wolf, K. (1933) Anstaltspfledge und Entwicklung im ersten Lebensjahar. *Zeitschrift für kinder forschung*, 42/3.

Eisenberg, L. (1964) Behavioural manifestations of cerebral damage in childhood. In H. G. Birch (Ed.) *Brain damage in children.* Baltimore: Williams & Wilkins.

Eysenck, H. J. (1968a) *The biological basis of personality.* Springfield: Thomas.

Eysenck, H. J. (1968b) A dimensional system of psychodiagnostics. In A. R. Mahrer (Ed.) *New approaches to psychodiagnostic systems.* New York: Aldine.

Eysenck, H. J. & Eysenck, S. B. G. (1969) Psychoticism in children: a new personality variable. *Res. in Education*, 1, 21–37.

Fantz, R. L. (1967) Visual perception and experience in early infancy. A look at the hidden side of behaviour development. In H. W. Stevenson, E. H. Hess & H. L. Rheingold (Eds.) *Early behaviour comparative and developmental approaches.* New York: Wiley.

Fairweather, D. V. & Illsley, R. (1960) Obstetric and social origins of mentally handicapped children. *Brit. J. Prev. Soc. Med.*, 14, 149–159.

Hardman, K. (1970) Motor impairment and socialisation. Unpublished paper, Dept. of Physical Education, Leeds University.

Hewett, S., Newson, J. & Newson, E. (1970) *The family and the handicapped child.* London: Allen & Unwin.

Jones, M. C. & Bayley, N. (1950) Physical maturing among boys as related to behaviour. *J. Educ. Psych.*, 41, 129–148.

Kaupe, W. (1920) Hospitalismes der in säughlingsheimen untergebrachten kindern. *Munchen med. Wohnschr.*, No. 8.

Knobloch, H. & Pasamanick, B. (1959) The syndrome of minimal cerebral damage in infancy. *J.A.M.A.*, 170, 1384–1387.

Lilienfeld, A. M., Pasamanick, B. & Rogers, M. (1955) Relationships between pregnancy experience and the development of certain neuro-psychiatric disorders in childhood. *Am. J. Public Health*, 45, 637–643.

Montague, M. F. A. (1950) Constitutional and prenatal factors in infant child health. In G. Newton & S. Levine (Eds.) *Early experience and behaviour.* Springfield: Thomas.

Northway, M. L. (1966) Unpublished lecture, London University, Institute of Education.

Oseretzky, N. A. (1929) A group method of examining the motor functions of children and adolescents. *Z. Kinderfersch*, 35, 332–372.

Osgood, C. E. & Sebeck, T. A. (Eds.) (1954) *Psycho-linguistics—A survey of theory and research problems.* Indiana: University Press.

Pasamanick, B., Rogers, M. E. & Lilienfeld, A. M. (1956) Pregnancy experience and development of behaviour disorder in children. *Am. J. Psychiat.*, 112, 613–618.

Prechtl, H. F. R. (1961) Neurological sequelae of pre-natal and para-natal complications. In B. Foss (Ed.) *Determinants of infant behaviour*, I. London: Methuen.

Prechtl, H. F. R. (1963) The mother-child interaction in babies with minimal brain damage. In B. Foss (Ed.) *Determinants of infant behaviour*, II. London: Methuen.

Radin, N. & Sonquist, H. (1968) Ypsilanti public schools Gale pre-school program. Cyclostyled final report (from the authors).

Richardson, S. A. (1964) The social environment and individual functioning. In H. G. Birch (Ed.) *Brain damage in children: the biological and social aspects*. New York: Williams & Wilkins.

Rogers, M., Lillienfeld, A. M. & Pasamanick, B. (1955) Prenatal and paranatal factors in the development of childhood behaviour disorders. *Acta Psychiat. et Neur.*, Scand. Supplement No. 102.

Schaffer, H. R. (1965) Changes in developmental quotient under two conditions of maternal separation. *Brit. J. Soc. Clin. Psych.*, 4, 39–46.

Schaffer, H. R. (1966) Activity level as a constitutional determinant of infantile reaction to deprivation. *Child Dev.*, 37, 3, 592–602.

Schaffer, H. R. & Emerson, P. E. (1968) The effects of experimentally administered stimulation on developmental quotients of infants. *Brit. J. Soc., Clin. Psych.*, 7, 61–67.

Silver, A. A. (1958) Behavioural syndrome associated with brain damage in children. *Paedriatric Clinics of North America*, 6, 687–698.

Skinner, B. F. (1953) *Science and human behaviour*. New York: Macmillan.

Stevenson, H. W. (1965) Social reinforcement in children's behaviour. In R. H. Walters & R. D. Parkes (Eds.) *Advances in child development and behaviour*, 2. New York: Academic Press.

Stott, D. H. (1959) *Unsettled children and their families*. London: University Press.

Stott, D. H. (1962) Evidence for a congenital factor in maladjustment and delinquency. *Am. J. Psych.*, 118, 781–794.

Stott, D. H. (1964) Why maladjustment? *New Society*, Dec. 10th.

Stott, D. H. (1966) *Studies of troublesome children*. London: Tavistock.

Strauss, A. A. & Kephart, N. C. (1955) *Psychopathology and education of the brain-injured child*. New York: Grave & Stratton.

Sutton-Smith, B. & Roberts, J. M. (1964) Rubrics of competitive behaviour. *J. Gen. Psych.*, 105, 13–37.

Talbot, F. (1941) Transactions of the American Pediatric Society —discussion of paper by Bakwin. *Am. J. Dis. Child.*, 62, 469.

Walters, R. H. & Parke, R. D. (1964) Social maturation, dependency and susceptibility to social influence. In L. Berkowitz (Ed.) *Advances in experimental social psychology*, 1. New York: Academic Press.

Whiting, H. T. A., Morris, P. R., Davies, J. G., Gibson, J. M., Lumley, R. & Sutcliffe, R. S. E. (1970) Motor impairment in an approved school population. Unpublished paper, Dept. of Physical Education, Leeds University.

CHAPTER 5

Body Concept

Genetic psychology makes it clear that the infant is not a self, a personality. He is only a kind of candidate for personality. If he attains it in some measure, he does so gradually. It is an achievement, not a gift. Neither is it the necessary and inevitable unfolding of powers within him. It is actually developed through concrete and vital experiences, or if these experiences do not occur, it is not developed at all. It is just as true, therefore, to say that one gets the idea of himself from the objects he deals with, and that he makes them the pattern upon which he constructs the self, as it is to say that the reverse occurs.

(Ames, 1910)

An increasing concern with the 'body concept' by workers in the field of compensatory education is reflected in a wide variety of studies. Benyon (1968) for example, reporting on intensive programming for slow-learners lists the fundamental areas of weakness in children referred to her clinic as:

1. Body image
2. Position in space
3. Form constancy
4. Sensory integration

and at the same time appreciates that such areas are far from being independent of one another. The 6–8-year-old children concerned were referred to the clinic because they were unable to read, write or do arithmetic; speech and language were deficient; following simple directions was inconsistent and discipline and emotional problems apparent.

It is interesting to note Benyon's description of body-image as:

an overall concept of one's body and its movements with relationship to varied environments

what she refers to as a 'workable body image' reflecting the way in which the individual is able to integrate his responses to the demands of the environment—an integration of input and output information. An operationally defined limited body-image is apparent in Benyon's observations of children attending the clinic:

> Each child was 'insecure' with himself; he was not aware of what, where or who he was or exactly how he was functioning with relation to his environment. His body often baffled him as it got him into constant trouble by bumping into things, tripping over itself, getting 'lost' in clothing, and failing to allow him to ride bikes, climb trees, or play ball like any of his friends. He also found himself forgetting about his body often acting on impulse with total disregard for the consequences.

Terminology

Variations in terminology and emphasis by different writers on the theme of 'body-concept' make precise definitions difficult to come by. The operational definition of Benyon is perhaps more meaningful within the present context. The fact that the description she gives fits the idea of clumsiness expounded in this book makes the question of body-image central to the problem of compensatory education. The term 'body-image' is probably the most utilised in the literature although the ambiguity implicit in the term will be apparent from the following brief comment on some of its usages.

Schilder (1935), a German neurologist, was one of the earlier writers on this topic. He discusses the concept in the following way:

> The body schema is the tridimensional image everybody has about himself. We may call it 'body image'. The term indicates that we are not dealing with a mere sensation or imagination. There is a self-appearance of the body . . . there are mental pictures and representations involved in it, but it is not mere representation.

Although nothing is said explicitly about the way in which such an image will affect performance, it seems reasonable to suppose that such a schema will be an important mediating process in relation to bodily actions. The terminology, however, is still vague and lacking in precision. In the terms used, it clearly overlaps the usage of concepts like ego, self and self-concept (Fisher & Cleveland, 1958). Such an overlap is further reflected in Wright's (1960) description of the body-image as:

> . . . that aspect of the self-concept which pertains to attitudes and experiences involving the body.

Fenichel (1945) is more explicit:

> . . . the sum of the mental representations of the body and its organs, the so-called body-image constitutes the idea of I and is of basic importance for the further formation of the ego.

Although some of the evidence on which 'body-image' develops is—according to the sources discussed—obtained as the result of feedback from the individual's own movement behaviour and is in consequence somehow more personal, the idea of an effective value-loaded concept of the body implies interaction with others. This kind of approach is reflected in Witkin *et al.*'s (1962) coining of the term 'body-concept' representing:

> The systematic impression an individual has of his body, cognitive and affective, conscious and unconscious formed in the process of growing up.

This to Witkin *et al.* arises out of the full gamut of his experiences with his own body and the bodies of others in the course of development. While the experimental work of Witkin and his colleagues has been primarily concerned with the global body-concept, a number of his contemporaries (Werner, Wapner & Canali, 1957; Liebert, Werner & Wapner, 1958; Humphries, 1959; Wapner, McFarland & Werner, 1962) became interested in the 'body boundary'—the differentiation of self from environment. Merleau-Ponty (1962) sees the development of such differentiation to be an important aspect of perceptual development and does not really delineate— at least in developmental terms—between 'body-boundary' and 'body-image' except to suggest that realisation of the former is necessary for the latter. In this respect, it is worth being reminded that the skin forms the ultimate body-boundary and it is at this interface between body and external environment that exchange of information takes place.

A concern with the 'translatory' characteristics (Chapter 1) of 'body-image' is apparent in Ritchie-Russell's (1958) definition of the 'body-image system' as:

> . . . that which makes it possible for appropriate bodily movements to be performed in relation to afferent stimuli.

An intact 'body-image system' is necessary for such appropriate actions to take place—there must be an awareness of the position of the body in space. Any deficit may affect the ability of the child to fulfil the most basic functions of walking, feeding, dressing and washing.

The 'body-concept' is extended even further in the physical education literature where the term 'body-awareness' is often encountered. Although seldom clearly defined, there is a tendency with some writers to equate the term 'body-awareness' with 'general kinesthetic sensitivity'. Now, while most of the writers already quoted would be willing to agree that kinesthetic information plays some part in development of the 'body-concept', other sources of information are considered to be of some importance. While it is possible to define 'body-awareness' in terms of a *general* sensitivity to kinesthetic information, it is not clear that this is a particularly meaningful approach. Dickinson (1970) has drawn attention to the limitations implicit in a definition of this kind and quoted research evidence for the relatively *specific* nature of the kinesthetic sense modalities.

Within this brief-overview, the body-concept in a variety of terms has been associated by different writers with:

(a) the ability to make body movements appropriate to the demands of the environment
(b) bodily sensations
(c) imagination—mental imagery which is not purely representational
(d) ego-development
(e) affective-development
(f) cognitive-development
(g) the development of body-boundaries
(h) kinesthetic sensitivity

All these possibilities would seem to be of significance in relation to compensatory education but dealing with such an all-embracing concept is difficult. Argyle (1969) reflects this difficulty in suggesting that:

> Body-image in certain respects overlap the various usages of concepts like ego, self and self-phenomenon relating to attitudes towards the body, it has wider implications which cross-over into other personality areas.

Without at this stage becoming involved in the development of the 'self' which has much wider implications than can be dealt with in a single chapter, it is worth noting Argyle's (1969) differentiation between two aspects of the 'self':

1. 'I'—the conscious subject—the decision-maker
2. 'Me'—reacted to by others as being a particular sort of person. Such reactions give rise within the individual to concepts of:

   (a) self-image—referring to the perception of the person by himself—what sort of person he thinks he is in a descriptive way.
   (b) self-esteem—how favourably he regards himself.

Between them they form a cognitive system which like other cognitive systems exerts a controlling effect on behaviour.

Body-image within such a framework would be classified as part of the self-image.

'Body-concept' and information processing
In discussing the inaccuracy of Morison's (1969) concept of 'body-awareness', Dickinson (1970) has suggested that the concept should be reinterpreted in terms of present theories of attention. It is suggested that such an idea should be extended to the 'body-concept' in general as discussed in the chapter so far.

In terms of the information-processing model presented in Chapter 1 it will be appreciated that information from the external environment which is not the result of the individual's own actions (exafferent) together with reafferent information (which is the result of his own actions) will contribute towards the development of the 'body-concept'. The establishment of such a conceptual framework within the memory systems reflecting both cognitive and affective information will serve as a mediating mechanism between stimulus and response. A reciprocal relationship would appear to exist. Information from the internal and external environment leads to a build-up of the 'body-concept' and the presence of such a frame of reference leads to a more selective information intake from the environment. Meredith (1966) makes the same point in a different context:

> It is as true to say that the hand controls the brain as that the brain controls the hand—in the sense that the hand has evolved as the primary executive organ for grasping, exploring and responding to the environment, a physical mediator of compulsions. For it is the *events* in the brain which are all-important and these are in part the resultants of events all over the body. The viewpoint to be defined here directs us to approach our task of interpretation as that of giving functional significance to elaborate and widely distributed systems of neural events.

Wober (1966) in a novel approach to the study of 'body-concept' has coined the term 'sensotype' which implies a predisposition to attend to one class of input information rather than another. Thus, in some cultures more emphasis will be placed on proprioceptive information in development while in others the visual may be considered to be of primary importance. The resultant mediating mechanisms would lead to a bias towards a particular class of information. It seems possible that hierarchical systems of selection might also be established. This would be consistent with the effects of experience on the development of particular perceptual analysers (Treisman, 1969). It is not clear to what extent primary emphasis on a particular class of sensory input will facilitate or handicap development within a particular culture and to what extent such a procedure will limit the transferability of an individual across cultures or to different task performances within a particular culture.

Biesheuvel (1963) has discussed the limitations imposed by lack of opportunity for learning particular skills in relation to African populations. He suggests that failure to provide the right psychomotor experience at particular maturational stages will prevent the full realisation of potential ability. While the maturational concept might be questioned, he does

raise the interesting proposition as to whether limited opportunities for learning certain basic movement habits in the tribal or
urban African environment may be responsible for the difficulties which Africans experience in acquiring the manual dexteri-
ties needed for certain skilled trades. The discrepancy which
exists between the performance of tribesmen and educated
white or African groups is illustrated in Figure 8 for a two hand
coordination task.

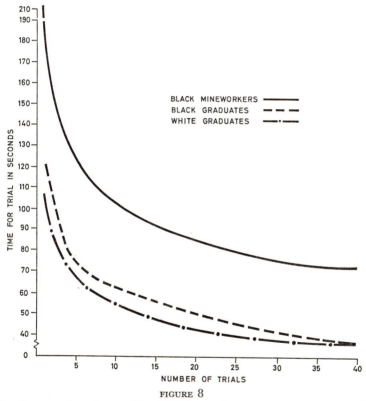

FIGURE 8

Psychomotor learning on Two Hand Coordination Test by White and
Black adults of different educational and cultural levels

Biesheuvel suggests that a *prima facie* case exists for providing
African children with more opportunity to manipulate, to
diversify their motor-responses and habits and to exercise these
basic skills more continually.

This problem is perhaps reflected in Abercrombie & Tyson's
(1966) discussion of the difficulties encounted in 'switching'

I

attention when particular modes of information processing are not clearly established. This may have considerable importance in developing compensatory education programmes for motor-impaired children particularly in relation to the concepts of hyperactivity and distractibility:

> The description of this 'troubled' behaviour resulting apparently from alternating attentiveness to positional or to musical cues are reminiscent of the behaviour of some cerebral palsied children. . . . It may be that, like Witkins' 'troubled' subjects, such children are alternating in attentiveness to the visual field at one moment and to their bodily sensations of the vertical at another.

This might well be conceived as an undeveloped 'differentiation' in Witkin et al.'s terms or be looked upon as an inability to discriminate between relevant and irrelevant sets of sub-threshold intensity signals in Dickinson's (1970) terms.

The linking of body-concept in one form or another with information processing is not a new idea. Fisher (1965) discusses body-image as a 'source of selective cognitive sets', suggesting that an individual's body experiences produce effects upon his cognitions. Studies such as those of Werner & Wapner (1952); McFarland (1958); Calloway & Dembro (1958) and Hinckley & Rethlingschafer (1951) have related level of muscle tonus, degree of autonomic arousal and body crippling to the reception and elaboration of particular stimuli. Helson (1958) also points out that bodily sensations contribute to the general adaptation level and hence have an influence on the way in which judgements are made.

In his paper, Fisher assumes that there are forms of bodily experience which serve as peristent signals to orient the individual to reception or rejection of certain classes of information. This has previously been referred to as 'selective attention'.

> It may be presumed that the patterns of body activation exist as circuits based on the following sequence: perceptual focus upon a body area because of its utility or significance or activation in relation to a goal, increased physiological and also sensory arousal of the area as a consequence of the special prominence, further feedback from such arousal to the subsystems in the C.N.S. involved in the initiation of the original highlighting of this area. Thus, the individual's

body scheme contains landmarks which reiterate to him that certain things are important and others are not.

In relation to the concept of 'arousal' the importance of kines-thetic feedback has been stressed by Bernhaut *et al.* (1953). They suggest that such information is more important than visual or auditory stimulation for reticular activation. Kulka *et al.* (1960) have proposed further that rocking and head bang-ing and other such rhythmic movements which are seen in infants with prolonged deprivation are attempts to gratify kinesthetic needs in arousal terms.

There are many reports in the literature of distortions of body-image from subjects undergoing sensory or perceptual deprivation situations. Francis (1968) summarises some of these findings as follows:

> There was a report of a feeling of lying on a bed and also that the lower part of the body was immobilised by being held. Another case reported an impression that someone was holding the legs and feet and in consequence the S could not move them. Yet another S reported that sensation from the lower part of the body was completely absent and another S reported a distinct impression that someone was in the pool beside him. The S kicked out at the intruder.

Head (1926) draws attention to the importance of moment to moment variations in postural experiences and the effect these may have on early development. The effects of limited ex-perience for discrimination and generalisation of such forms of sensory input in this respect will be appreciated.

An interpretation of these latter findings could probably be made in terms of the idea of 'signal/noise ratio' raised earlier in Chapter 1. It would be anticipated that the processing of unnecessary information about the body processes because of a failure (on the basis of past experience) to appreciate informa-tion which is relevant and information which is not, would lead to an increase of the 'noise' level in the cortex making dis-crimination of other—perhaps more important—information from other sources more difficult.

Selective attention has figured in Witkin's (1965) attempts to relate the degree of sophistication of body-concept to the mode of perceptual functioning termed field dependence/independence. Field independent perceivers are considered to have a relatively articulated impression of the body as distinct from its surrounding field and of the parts of the body as being separated but inter-related in a clear structure. Field independent perceivers can easily separate an item from its background, but field-dependent perceivers find this difficult and are slow to isolate particular items. This work will receive further consideration.

Development of the body-concept

Related to Witkin *et al.*'s (1962) concept of articulation is that of 'psychological differentiation'. The new-born baby probably experiences himself as a 'more or less continuous body-field matrix'. Although current findings on inter-uterine experience and Fantz's (1958) work on early infantile perceptual abilities would lead to caution in acceptance of James (1890) idea that such very young children experience the world as a 'blooming, buzzing confusion', any differentiation at this stage is likely to be very restricted and one view of development would be in terms of progress towards greater differentiation within the body-concept and body function. Thus, an original 'global' impression of the body should give rise to an awareness of the parts of the body, the way in which they interrelate and their potential for displacement within the environment. That is, towards differentiation of inner structure and function and towards an appreciation of spatial concepts such as 'top and bottom', 'back and front', 'right and left' in relation to the body as a frame of reference. An appreciation will be developed of the body as having definite limits or boundaries and of the parts within as being discrete yet interrelated (differentiation/ integration hypothesis) and joined in a definite structure (Witkin *et al.*, 1962).

The development of the body-concept cannot of course be divorced from the study of child development. Fisher & Cleveland (1958) reinforce what has been said above in suggesting that body-image development begins early in life and probably at about six months of age. Piaget (1952) as might be expected has given some attention to the body concept. He suggests that the development of the body-schema runs parallel with sensori-motor development reflecting once again the importance of movement activity with its related kinesthetic feedback.

Freud (1961) postulated a three-stage libido organisation theory in which the erogenic zones constitute the initial developmental areas of body-image development.

To Witkin *et al.* (1962) the development of a differentiation between self and field is a gradual process. The development of self is rooted in but not limited to, sensations generated by body functions and allied activities. It is rather more derived from all the experiences which a child encounters during development in relation to his own body and the body of others:

> Through experiencing pleasure or pain, success or failure, pride or shame in connection with the body and by incorporating the social values which the environment attaches to the body and its parts, the person's body-concept becomes heavily invested with a variety of special and highly personal meanings, feelings and values.

The importance of 'touch' in the development of differentiation and the establishment of body-boundaries should not be denigrated. A syndrome termed 'touch hunger' has been noted in relation to maladjusted children where the close-contact which normally exists between parents and offspring has been missed. Kydd (1962) in discussing this phenomenon elaborates on such a relationship:

> . . . take a close look at a really loving mother with her baby, and young children. They worship each other through their senses; they are in the grip of a passion almost sexual in its intensity and exclusiveness. Watch the mother stroking the baby's legs, listen to her descriptions of her four-year-old's strength and daring, watch the seven-year-old get comfort from merely holding his mother's hand. Notice, too, the place of the father, how important to a child is sitting on his father's knee, or playing those immemorial games that involve being thrown into the air and caught.

Aspects of development of this kind tend to be overlooked in relation to *normal* development. They make a bigger impression in relation to, for example, the education of blind children. In this respect the contribution made by touch to the education of people like Helen Keller cannot be over-emphasised.

It is surprising how an appreciation of the usefulness of non-verbal education pervades much of the writing of Huxley (1938) for example perhaps reflecting the influence of Eastern philosophy and its ideas on the training of awareness. The development of body-awareness is clearly related to the instruction 'know thyself'. As recently as 1961, Huxley returns to the same theme:

> Now it seems to me that we have to think of education also on the non-verbal level: we have to think of the possibility of training directly the mind-body that has to do the learning and the living. We don't do very much of this at present. We concentrate chiefly on the verbal level and don't do very much for the strange multiple amphibian organism which we possess. There is a very remarkable phrase which Spinoza uses, which seems all the more remarkable when one thinks of the extraordinary abstractness of his writings: he says 'Teach the body to do many things; this will help you to perfect the mind and to come to the intellectual level of thought'. I think it is a phrase of immense importance. If we substitute for the word 'body' the word 'organism' and for the word 'mind' the word 'mind-body', this could be made the motto of an entirely new branch of education, the deliberate training of the mind-body, which then has to make use of its concepts and its words.

Jourard (1967) has been particularly active in pointing out the limited use of touch within Western societies in particular. He suggests that there may be a connection between 'body experience' ('what someone perceives, believes, imagines, feels and fantasies about his body') and physical and mental health:

> It's almost as if all possible meanings of a touch are eliminated except the caress with sexually arousing intent. Not that there is anything wrong with the latter; but it does imply that unless a young American (or British?) adult is engaged in sexual lovemaking he is unlikely to experience his body as it feels when someone is touching, poking, massaging, hugging or holding it.

He points out that increasing numbers of psychotherapists are interesting themselves in techniques for awakening a benumbed body consciousness. A growing body of teachers of body awareness conduct classes aimed at undoing the repression of body experience.

While the importance of *particular* sensory systems in the development of body-image have not been emphasised, it *is* important to note possible differences. The importance of touch has just been commented upon. Allport (1957) points out that the body sense (coenaesthesis—stimuli from muscles, viscera, tendons joints and vestibular organs) is one of the first feedback systems to be encountered in the development of awareness. He considers that while coenaesthesis remains a lifelong anchor for self-awareness it never accounts for the entire sense of self.

Wober (1966) as already stated (page 86) has coined the term 'sensotype' to represent the pattern of relative importance of the different senses by which a child learns to perceive the world and in which pattern his abilities develop. Within different cultures, it is not surprising to find that emphasis on particular modes of information processing should differ. He reports individual differences in a Nigerian population in relation to their cognitive and analytic approach to perceived material:

> It is possible to interpret these results in terms of an elaboration of skills and analytic functioning, not as a generalised phenomenon within each individual but related to particular fields of sensory experience. That is to say the blind lacking a visual word would develop their differentiation and analytic abilities in an auditory world.

He found in such cultures an emphasis on proprioceptive and auditory information rather than visual and suggests that such a 'sensotype' is different from that of an individual skilled in the visual world. Jourard (1967) has also drawn attention to cross-cultural differences in the use of touch as a means of communication and contact.

The effects of early experience on development of the body-concept are reflected in observations made by Dyk & Witkin (1965) in a study relating family experiences to development of differentiation in children. Possible sources for a small but consistent sex difference was noticed in their performance on perceptual tests. There was an indication that mothers may have different emphasis in bringing up sons and daughters; mothers tending to be less accepting of assertiveness in their daughters and placing more emphasis on social skills. It was also noticed that daughters seemed to be reared in ways similar to those found among field-dependent boys. It was concluded that parental influences—particularly at an early age—do affect the development of the body-concept. Earlier (page 110) it was suggested that parents' attitudes towards the behaviour of their motor-impaired children might influence their social development. In the present context, it might be supposed that a similar effect might occur in relation to the development of the body-concept particularly in relation to the affective domain.

Body-concept and compensatory education

Kephart (1960) was one of the earlier workers in the field of compensatory education to realise the value of perceptual-motor training on integrated development. In particular, he emphasised the relationship between the development of body-image, the development of lateral and directional awareness and feedback in perception to learning disabilities.

The concept of laterality as an aspect of body-image has been considered to be critical in a motor hypothesis of school achievement but results have not been clear-cut. O'Connor (1969) for example in comparing the effects of a traditional physical education programme and physical activities in the form suggested by Kephart (1960) on motor, perceptual and academic achievement of first graders reported in favour of the Kephart method for measures of motor ability and internal lateral awareness. No significant differences were found between the two methods on measures of academic achievement, external lateral awareness, lateral preference or ability to draw geometric figures.

Hill *et al.* (1967) investigated the effect of a systematic programme of exercises on the development of retarded children's awareness of right-left directionality. In conclusion, these workers suggested that programmes for training retarded children should include activities which give them many experiences in orientating their attention to the position of their own bodies in space relative to that of other objects as well as directing children to make responses with specified body parts. Tansley (1967) repeats the message in reporting on the education of neurologically abnormal children whose difficulties lie in three main areas of dysfunction.

1. abnormal neurological development
2. perceptual disturbance
3. language dysfunction

In the particular experimental school with which his report

is concerned, training is given in such things as eye-hand coordination, form perception, visual discrimination, movement training of both a specific and of a more generalised nature. The latter being particularly concerned with improvement in the child's 'body-image'. Both encouraging and spectacular results are reported in the cognitive development of these children. Tansley also speculates:

> . . . one further exciting prospect is before us if all children could receive an early education based on similar rationale and practice, could the general levels of intelligence and achievement be raised significantly?

An important point in compensatory education programmes which is often missed, is that of integrating all phases of a particular programme. Radin & Sonquist (1968) reporting on the Gale pre-school programme give examples of such integration in stating that within the programme when the children worked at classifying two sizes they were encouraged to use sentences practised in the language programme, i.e. 'These plates are big and these plates are little'. Not only were such kinds of integration attempted, but the children were considered to be undergoing the programme the whole time they were in contact with the teacher or the aide. Thus:

> In outdoor activities, at wash-up time, and even lining up for the bathroom, the curriculum was in use. The teacher would not merely ask the children to put away the blocks, but to put the big blocks on the shelf for big blocks and the small blocks on the shelf for small blocks. When the children were called to sit at the table for juice, they were often not called by name but by the picture of the symbol each child had been assigned . . . at the juice table the opportunity was used to compare the cookies for work in spatial relation.

Psychologists such as Hostler (1966) would refer to some of these procedures as 'play with a purpose'. Motives other than pure enjoyment would seem to be involved. The question which arises is to whom the 'play' has a purpose—the child performing or the person structuring the situation or materials for play? If it is intended to impose purpose from the outside, should this in fact be made explicit to the child? Does the skill of the teacher lie in his ability to structure situations—including play

—for explicit purposes which both achieve these ends and gain the cooperation of the child?

Humphrey (1966) could be said to have used this approach in exploring the use of *active* games in the learning of number concepts by children. Games were those associated with pleasurable active experience. He draws attention to the important role played by kinesthetic feedback produced by body movement (reafference) although it is doubtful if his investigation really supports such an hypothesis. The same worker (Humphrey, 1965) also compared the use of active games and language workbook exercises as learning media in the development of language and understanding with children. While the children learned through both media, the active games group were superior.

Schilder (1935) puts the 'body-image' in a more fundamental position:

> . . . when the knowledge of our own body is incomplete or faulty all actions for which this particular knowledge is necessary will be faulty. We need the body-image in order to start movements.

He further points out that a fault in the body-image will be reflected in the perception of outside objects and that in order for a child to develop a reliable and consistent point of origin for perceptions and motor responses it is necessary for him to have a clear and concise concept of his body-image. Thus reiterating the input and output functions of a developed body-image.

Various modalities are involved in establishing the body-image. If one area of perceptual input is defective (as in blindness or deafness) an attempt must be made to compensate via other sensory modalities. As Stephenson & Robertson (1965) point out, when the handicap is severe—as in cerebral palsy—children must be assisted in using all the experience they can get. They suggest encouraging such children to roll and crawl, to feel their own bodies and to be aware of all their movements.

> The aim is not to teach the form of the body but to provide basic experience from which the concept can develop.

The spatial aspects of body-image have been stressed by Freedman (1961) in pointing out that the normal adult seems to structure his world in accordance with some overall spatial schema, depending upon various coordinations such as up-down, left-right, self-other. Distortions of a temporary kind will affect the person's orientation and failure to build-up an appropriate schema would be expected to lead to difficulties in spatial orientation. As Francis (1968) indicates, transactions with the environment require adequate localisation in the schema. There is an inter-dependence between body and spatial schema such that alteration of one produces changes in the other. He makes the further and often missed point that the body schema requires *continual maintenance* and this is effected by constant sampling of the environment. Deprivation situations would on this basis be expected to lead to distortion of body-image and if occurring in early stages of development limit the elaboration of such an image.

The concept of spatial schema is a difficult one to fully appreciate. Gibson (1966) has discussed this in a particularly meaningful way:

> Completely empty space is imperceivable. There are dimensions or axes of empty space to be sure but they are embodied in a solid environment having a north-south, an east-west and an up-down. This is the space to which an individual is oriented, with respect to which the posture and equilibrium of his body is maintained. The body itself, with its main axes of right-left, front-back and head-foot, must never be confused with it. I called this a 'vector space' on an earlier page but it is not really a space. The body percept, or 'body image' is a set of possible dispositions or poses— standing or lying—relative to the substratum and to gravity. If it is a space at all, it is subjective rather than objective. And it is fluid instead of rigid for it can adopt any of a vast family of poses by moving from one to another.

The interrelationship of body image and compensatory education is not a particularly new idea. It was implicit in the early work of Schilder (1935) and as long ago as 1932, Alexander (1957) suggested that by his procedures:

> a gradual improvement will be brought about in the pupil's sensory appreciation so that he will become more aware of faults in his habitual manner of using himself, correspondingly as with the increasing awareness of the manner of his use of himself improves, his sensory appreciation will further

improve and in time constitute a standard within the self by means of which he will become increasingly aware both of faults and improvement not only in the manner of his use but also in the standard of his functioning generally.

Huxley (1938) also speculated on the same problem in enlarging his concept of the principle of 'non-attachment'. To him, a good physical education should:

> ... teach awareness on the physical plane—not the obsessive and unwished for awareness that pain imposes upon the mind, but voluntary and intentional awareness. The body must be trained to think. . . . The awareness that our bodies need is the knowledge of some general principle of right integration and along with it, a knowledge of the proper way to apply that principle in every phase of mental activity.

Three further studies are worth quoting in relation to compensatory education as they raise points which need to be elaborated in later discussion. Painter (1964) for example carried out a study on the effect of rhythmic and sensory motor activities on the perceptual-motor-spatial abilities of kindergarten school children hypothesising that such a programme would be especially effective for those children with distortions in the concept of body-image. Using the Goodenough Draw-a-man test as a measure of a child's body-image concept (Witkin et al., 1962) she found that after such a programme there was indeed a marked improvement in the level of ability to draw a figure and thus an improvement in the distortion of a child's image. A similar method of assessment was utilised by Holden (1962) in attempting to determine whether summer camp experience had any effect on the body-image of physically handicapped children. It was hypothesised and confirmed that motor activities engaged in during a camping programme would enhance the child's awareness of his own body and this would be reflected in an improvement in human figure drawing.

These two studies highlight the difficulties involved in assessing body-image. Direct evidence of the nature of an individual's body-concept is difficult to obtain. The medium used most frequently is that of human figure drawing, here the subject is required to draw a person, and then a person of the opposite sex. The drawings are then scored against a sophistication of body-concept scale. The classification system in the Hanna Marlens rating scale (Witkin *et al.*, 1962) utilises a detailed definition of three categories of characteristics—form level, identity and sex differentiation and level of detail. From this scale rating a single rating based on both drawings is assigned to each subject.

In this brief overview, attention has been drawn to the importance attached to the concept of body-image in developmental and impairment studies. Hobbs (1966) has summed up the position:

> We are intrigued by the idea that the physical self is the armature around which the psychological self is constructed and that a clearer experiencing of the potential and the boundaries of the body should lead to a clearer definition of the self and thus to greater psychological fitness and more effective functioning.

Whether or not such a generalised improvement in performance is more than an act of faith, is open to question. Certainly those concerned with compensatory education of this kind should give heed to Doll's (1966) contention that 'there is a hint that through some occult process transfer of training occurs with generalised educational improvement in non-motor areas'. Evidence at the present time is limited for such a generality of transfer.

Assessing the body-concept
The 'draw-a-person' test has been the one most favoured in the literature for assessing the degree of sophistication of body-concept. Scoring is generally based on the Hanna Marlens scale (Witkin *et al.*, 1962).

There are difficulties with this kind of projective test. As Witkin *et al.* (1962) have suggested, such drawings like any other projective expression are obviously multi-determined. They suggest that the final product may represent:

> . . . in addition to the body concept itself, aspects of the broader self concept, a projection of the idealised self image, an expression of the concept of others in the environment, and it is influenced by cultural factors and by drawing skill as well.

Similar difficulties have been experienced in the use of the

Draw-a-man test to measure intelligence. For many years, studies of child development have been interested in the apparent relationship between children's maturing intellect and the progressively greater representation of detail and proportion which is shown in their drawings of the human person. In devising a scale to assess intelligence by means of children's drawings, Goodenough (1962) stressed several points:

1. Artistic standards were disregarded.
2. Efforts were made to eliminate subjective judgements as far as possible.
3. A standard subject for drawing was chosen but no other limitations were imposed.

The Goodenough scale now numbers fifty-one items, the norms being based upon the drawings of 2,306 children aged 4–10 years. Ansbacher (1952) studying 100 children with a mean age of 10 years, found that the Draw-a-man test correlated most highly with reasoning, spatial, perceptual factors and 'tracing'. It had least in common with verbal meaning and number.

In considering the relationships of the sophistication-of-body-concept scale with the Goodenough scale, Witkin et al. (1962) state:

> To a considerable extent, the two scales address themselves to similar aspects of figure drawings. The two scales relate similarly to perceptual index scores (0·53 for the Goodenough scale; 0·57 for the sophistication scale) and to total W.I.S.C. IQ (0·55 in both instances).

Oakley (1940) observed that with the coming of adolescence, drawings undergo considerable change and there is often a deterioration in quality: for example, lines are drawn indecisively and parts which are difficult to draw such as hands are sketchily treated or omitted. Oakley suggests that these changes come about through the child's losing confidence because he can now perceive how imperfect his drawings really are. Jones (1970) reports that many 19–20-year-old students in her study were well aware of their limited artistic ability and that scoring some of the drawings according to the sophistication of body-concept scale was very difficult. Nevertheless, she reports inter-scorer reliability coefficients of 0·66,

0·76 and 0·94 on a nine-point extension of the five-point Hanna Marlens scale.

Bearing the limitations of this procedure in mind, it is interesting to look at some of the efforts on this test by boys between the ages of 11·0 and 14·0 years attending a junior approved school (Whiting *et al.*, 1969). Figures 9–11 give some of the drawings together with shortened case histories.

Other means of assessing body-concept or aspects of it have been attempted from time to time. Fisher (1964) attempted to determine whether the stimulus character of the subject's own body may impinge upon learning and recall, or whether the prominence of the body in the perceptual field can affect a type of behaviour which is exemplified in learning and retention. In order to measure the prominence of the individual's own body, he based his results on the answer to the following question:

Write down 20 things you are conscious of right now.

The results were scored by summing the number of references that the subject made to himself. Fisher was here assuming that the greater the individual's perception was focused on his body, the more it should be mentioned.

His other test was to ask his subjects to look at a list of words: leg, house, car, thumb, toy, wrist, street, head, tent, skin, hammer, scooter, lever, book, hair, nose, glass, neck, hip, lamp. After one minute the list was removed and the subject asked to write down as many words as he could remember. The scoring method in this instance was to sum the 'body' words and subtract the 'non-body' words. A sample of ninety-two subjects produced results which significantly ($P < 0.001$) supported the hypothesis that the greater an individual's awareness of his own body in relation to his perceptual field, the more likely he is to display selectively superior recall for words referring to the body.

More recently, Stone (1968) investigating the relationships between the perception and reproduction of body postures used dynamic tests, and it is suggested that this might be a better medium in which to measure sophistication of body-concept. Jones (1970) has carried out pilot studies in this medium. Subjects were required to watch a movement sequence and then:

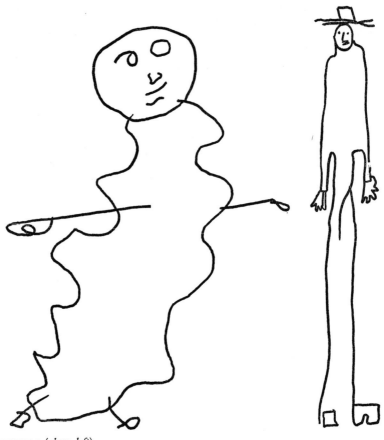

FIGURE 9 (*above, left*)
Case No. 19

Medical History: Pregnancy and birth normal.

Parents: Openly rejected by mother and father.

Reason for referral: Hyperkinetic autism diagnosed by psychiatrist at the hospital to whic parents took him. Extremely short span of attention—lapses into bouts of hand-rubbin; jumping up and down and rocking. Frequently drops things and knocks things ove Shows difficulty in walking and dexterous use of his hands.

FIGURE 10 (*above right*)
Case No. 20

Medical History: Normal pregnancy and birth. Two operations for removal of toenails ar an operation for rupture at 6½ years of age.

Mother: Married three times. Previous marriages ending in divorce. Recent treatment f acute depression.
 Stepfather has a good relationship with the boy.

Reason for referral: Uncontrollable, aggressive and destructive behaviour in and arour the home. No problem at school but lacked friends. A suggestion of a genetic predispositic to react adversely to stress.

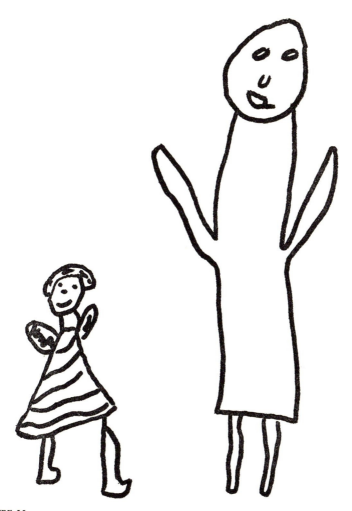

FIGURE II

Case No. 22

Medical History: Normal pregnancy and birth. Influenzal encephalitis at one year of age. Severe club feet necessitating a series of operations at four years of age.

Mother: A cheerful, bright person with a tendency to worry. No effective control over boy.

Reason for referral: Enuretic during day and night coupled with his being a constant source of trouble both at home and at school.

K

(*a*) perform it
(*b*) describe it on paper

Performances were scored according to the amount of body stress (as compared with space or effort stress) involved. In a further development, subjects watched a movement sequence based on body actions with particular stress on as many parts of the body as possible. They were asked to observe the bodily aspects of the movement and then:

(*a*) perform the sequence
(*b*) describe the sequence

Subjects were women students of physical education.

Further developments of this kind of approach to assessment are awaited with interest.

References

Abercrombie, M. L. J. & Tyson, M. C. (1966) Body image and draw-a-man test in cerebral palsy. *Dev. Med. Child Neur.*, 8, 9–15.

Alexander, F. M. (1957) *The use of the self.* London: Re-educational publication.

Allport, G. W. (1937) *Personality: a psychological interpretation.* New York: Holt.

Ames, E. S. (1910) *The psychology of religious experience.* New York: Cornwall.

Ansbacher, H. L. (1952) The Goodenough draw-a-man test and primary mental abilities. *J. Consult. Psych.*, 16, 176–180.

Argyle, M. (1969) *Social interaction.* London: Methuen.

Benyon, S. D. (1968) *Intensive programming for slow learners.* Ohio: Merrill.

Bernhaut, J. *et al.* (1953) Experimental contributions to the problem of consciousness. *J. Neurophysiol*, 16, 21–23.

Biesheuvel, S. (1963) The growth of abilities and character. *S. Afr. J. Sc.*, 59, 375–385.

Calloway, E. & Dembro, D. (1958) Narrowed attention: A psychological phenomenon that accompanies a certain physiological change. *Arch. neurol. Psychiat.*, 79, 74–90.

Dickinson, J. (1970) A note on the concept of body-awareness. *Brit. J. Phys. Educ.*, 1, 2, 34–36.

Doll, E. A. (1966) S.L.D. and motor training. *Percept. Motor Skills*, 23, 220.

Dyk, R. B. & Witkin, H. A. (1965) Family experiences related to the development of differentiation in children. *Child. Dev.*, 30, 1, 21–55.

Fantz, R. L. (1958) Pattern vision in young infants. *The Psych. Record*, 8, 43–47.

Fenichel, O. (1945) *The psychoanalytic theory of neurosis*. New York: Nortan.

Fisher, S. & Cleveland, R. L. (1958) *Body image and personality*. Princeton: Van Nostrand.

Fisher, S. (1964) Body awareness and selective memory for body versus non-body references. *J. Pers.*, 32, 138–144.

Fisher, S. (1965) The body-image as a source of selective cognitive sets. *J. of Pers.*, 33, 4, 536–552.

Francis, R. D. (1968) A conative hypothesis. *Bull. Brit. Psych. Soc.*, 21, 241–244.

Freedman, S. J. (1961) Sensory deprivation: Facts in search of a theory. *J. Nerv. Ment. Dis.*, 132, 17–21.

Freud, S. (1961) The ego and the id. In *Collected Works*, Vol. 19, London: Hogarth.

Gibson, J. J. (1966) *The senses considered as perceptual systems*. London: Allen & Unwin.

Goodenough, F. L. (1926) Measurement of intelligence by drawings. New York: Yonkerson-Hudson.

Head, H. (1926) *Aphasia and kindred disorders of speech*. London: Cambridge University Press.

Helson, H. (1958) The theory of adaptation-level. In D. C. Beardslee & M. Wertheimer (Eds.) *Readings in perception*. Princeton: Van Nostrand.

Hill, S. D. *et al.* (1967) Relation of training in motor activity to development of right-left directionality in mentally retarded children. *Percept. & Motor Skills*, 24, 363–366.

Hinckley E. D. & Rethlingschafer, D. (1951), Value judgements of heights of men by college students. *J. Psych.*, 31, 257–262.

Hobbs, N. (1966) Helping disturbed children: psychological and ecological strategies. *American Psych.*, 21, 12, 1105–1115.

Holden, R. H. (1962) Changes in the body-image of physically handicapped children due to summer day-camp experience. *Merill-Palmer Quarterly*, 8, 19–26.

Hostler, P. (1966) Play with a purpose. In *The world of children*. London: Paul Hamlyn.

Humphries, O. (1959) Effect of articulation of finger tip through touch on apparent length of outstretched arms. M.A. thesis, Clark University, Worcester, Mass.

Humphrey, J. H. (1965) Comparison of the use of active games and language work book exercises. *Percept. & Motor Skills*, 21, 23–26.

Humphrey, J. H. (1966) An exploratory study of active games in learning of number concepts. *Percept. & Motor Skills*, 23, 341–342.

Huxley, A. (1938) *Ends and means.* London: Chatto & Windus.

Huxley, A. (1961) Human potentialities. In S. M. Farber & R. H. L. Wilson (Eds.) *Control of the Mind.* New York: McGraw-Hill.

James, W. (1890) *Principles of psychology.* New York: Holt, Rinehart & Winston.

Jones, M. G. (1970) Perception, personality and movement. M.Ed. thesis, University of Leicester, England.

Jourard, S. (1967) Out of touch: the body taboo. *New Society*, 9.

Kulka, A., Fry, C. & Goldstein, F. J. (1960) Kinesthetic needs in infancy. *Amer. J. Orthopsychiat.*, 30, 306–314.

Kephart, N. C. (1960) *The slow learner in the classroom.* Ohio: Merrill.

Kydd, R. (1962) Touch hunger. In R. Johnson (Ed.) *An ABC of behaviour problems*, Vol. 10. Magazine of the Residential Child Care Association.

Liebert, R. S., Werner, H. & Wapner, S. (1958) Studies in the effect of lysergic acid diethylamide; self and object size perception in schizophrenic and normal adults. *A. M. A. Arch., Neur., Psychiat.*, 79, 580–584.

McFarland, J. H. (1958) The effect of a symmetrical muscular involvement on visual clarity. Paper presented at East. Psych. Ass. New York.

Meredith, P. (1966) *Instruments of communication.* London: Pergamon.

Merleau-Ponty, M. (1962) *Phenomenology of perception.* London: Routledge & Kegan Paul.

Morison, R. (1969) *A movement approach to educational gymnastics.* London: Dent.

Oakley, C. A. (1940) Drawings of a man by adolescents. *Brit. J. Psych.*, 31, 37–60.

O'Connor, C. (1969) Effects of selected physical activities upon motor performance, perceptual performance and academic achievement of first graders. *Percept. & Motor Skills*, 29, 703–709.

Painter, G. B. (1964) The effect of rhythmic and sensory motor activity programs on perceptual-motor-spatial abilities of kindergarten children. M.S. thesis, University of Illinois.

Piaget, J. (1952) *The origins of intelligence in children*, New York: International Press.

Radin, N. & Sonquist, A. (1968) Ypsilanti Public Schools—Gale preschool program. Mimeographed report (from authors).

Ritchie-Russell, W. (1958) Disturbance of the body-image. *Cerebral Palsy Bull.*, 4, 7–9.

Schilder, P. (1935) *The image and appearance of the human body.* London: Kegan Paul.

Stephenson, E. & Robertson, J. (1965) Normal child development and handicapped children. In J. G. Howells (Ed.) *Modern perspectives in child psychiatry.* Edinburgh: Oliver & Boyd.

Stone, R. E. (1968)   Relation between the perception and reproduction of body postures. *Res. Quart.*, 39, 3, 721–727.

Tansley, M. E. (1967)   The education of neurologically abnormal children. *Times Educ. Suppl.*, Jan. 20th.

Treisman, A. (1969)   Strategies and models of selective attention. *Psych. Rev.*, 76, 3, 282–299.

Wapner, S., McFarland, J. H. & Werner, H. (1962)   The effect of postural factors on the distribution of tactual sensitivity and the organisation of tactual kinesthetic space. *J. Exp. Psych.*, 63, 148–154.

Werner, H. & Wapner, S. (1952)   Toward a general theory of perception. *Psych. Rev.*, 59, 324–338.

Werner, H., Wapner, S. & Canali, P. E. (1957)   Effect of boundary on perception of head size. *Percept. & Motor Skills*, 7, 69–71.

Whiting, H. T. A., Davies, J. G., Gibson, J. M., Lumley, R., Sutcliffe, R. S. E. & Morris, P. R. (1969)   Motor-impairment in an approved school population. Unpublished paper. Dept. of Physical Education, Leeds University.

Witkin, H. A., Dyk. R. B., Faterson, D. R. & Karp, S. A. (1962)   *Psychological differentiation*. New York: Wiley.

Witkin, H. A. (1965)   Psychological differentiation and forms of pathology. *J. Abn. Psych.*, 70, 5.

Wober, M. (1966)   Sensotypes. *J. Soc. Psych.*, 70, 181–189.

Woods, G. E. (1958)   The development of body image. *Cerebral Palsy Bull.*, 4, 9–17.

Wright, B. A. (1960)   *Physical disability—a psychological approach.* New York: Harper & Row.

CHAPTER 6

Assessing Motor Impairment

The whole enterprise of psychometrics has been devoted to measuring what are regarded as objective, genetically fixed quantities, instead of pursuing a constructive aim to ascertain what can be done to improve labile, educationally plastic capacities for mental growth.

(Meredith, 1964)

A consideration of the possible causes

Since the suggestion has already been made that the difficulties that many children encounter in skill learning and performance may be attributed to the effects of neural dysfunction or minimal brain damage it would seem logical that a test of brain damage would be the most appropriate means of diagnosing the main cause of motor impairment. There is some doubt, however, that such an examination would be sufficiently sensitive to be able to detect the minor degrees of damage that may be involved. The question must also be considered as to the practical value of such diagnosis in assisting with any remediation or compensatory education that may be possible. In this respect a knowledge of the root cause of impairment in which damage to the brain is involved would appear to be almost incidental.

In order to be of any practical use the information obtained from a diagnostic test of minimal brain damage must be related to the effects of the damage as they become manifest in the learning difficulties of the individual.

Any test that may be used in the identification of children who are motor impaired must be concerned with the responses of the individual in respect of the tasks that he is required to perform as part of the everyday activities in his life. The selection of test items, based upon this criteria, will therefore be determined by cultural and other factors such as the age, sex, level of maturation and environmental background of the individual. The extent of the problem can only be measured in terms of these individual circumstances and not by any universal standards of performance. As mentioned in the Introduction it is a problem which, in a sense, has been created by the demands made upon the individual to learn certain skills that are regarded as important or at least desirable from an educational point of view.

Difficulties of identification

By a changing emphasis away from conformity, contemporary methods in education have, to a certain extent, alleviated this aspect of the problem. Unfortunately the effect of abolishing prescribed patterns of skilled behaviour only eliminates the actual and not the potential 'failures'. In addition, the removal of these standards has made it increasingly difficult for the teacher or other observer to make an objective assessment of a child's deficiencies. Clearly, therefore, there is a need to establish a reliable test or other procedure that can be applied in schools as a 'screening device' for the initial identification of children who have difficulty in learning and performing simple everyday skills.

On the basis of this criterion a test that included a selection of the 'important and desirable skills' would appear, at first sight, to be an appropriate line of approach. Unfortunately, it would be impossible to include all of the many different factors involved in the performance of motor skills in a limited number of items. The wide range of individual differences in abilities, interests and previous learning, etc., involves an unmanageable number of variables. The fact of the specificity of skills and skill learning would be sufficient reason to doubt the validity of any small sample. It would therefore be incorrect to assume that every child who was unable to perform a few selected skills was impaired. In addition, any assessment of performance on the basis of a pass or fail reflects more such factors as the opportunity for, and extent of, previous practice than the actual capabilities of a child.

It may be argued that the teacher's rating of a child's

capabilities and short-comings, made with the knowledge of his background, attitude to work, and other relevant factors, would provide a more accurate assessment of the situation. With access to a child's school records showing his progress and standards of achievement in the various subjects, a teacher may obtain a relatively clear indication of a child's specific learning difficulties. The value of this source of information was acknowledged by Cruickshank and his colleagues (1961) who commented upon the following sample of information obtained from achievement-test results:

> Wide discrepancies, for example, between language and non-language scores, failure to discriminate between similarities and differences, and evidence of right-left confusion are, as most teachers are aware, general guides in identifying the strengths and weaknesses of a given child in terms of his potential for achievement when compared with the strengths, weaknesses and achievement level of classmates of the same chronological age.
>
> The subtest score profile of under-achieving children, if properly understood, acts as a clue to developmental differences and deviations.

There is little doubt that this type of information would be extremely valuable in any diagnosis of the possible reasons why a particular child had difficulty in performing certain skills. The reliability of this assessment alone as a screening device must be closely examined for a wide discrepancy undoubtedly exists in any subjective observations by teachers or parents. The criteria upon which these judgements are based will vary according to the different views of normality and different standards of performance which are relative to each set of circumstances. In spite of this discrepancy the opinions of the teacher and perhaps those of an observant parent are the only means that operate at the moment for identifying children who are motor impaired.

Although a teacher may observe a certain lack of coordination or control, and he may be aware that a number of children appear to be incapable of performing even the simple skills such as catching a ball or skipping with a rope, there are no means at his disposal which may direct him in the important task of helping the children to overcome their difficulties.

It is important therefore in the formulation of any programme of compensatory education to find out what the difficulties are, and the manner and extent to which they may handicap educational development. If it is accepted that, in the first instance, some means of identification is necessary, either by teacher's assessment and/or some form of standardised test, then the next stage would appear to be a diagnostic test involving motor responses. It would be hoped that this would provide some usable information, not necessarily about the cause, but about the 'reasons why' some children are unable to perform certain skills effectively.

From the point of view of treatment, it is important that such diagnosis is made as early as possible as it becomes increasingly difficult with advancing age. Although a certain amount of compensation for any neuromotor disability takes place during the process of maturation, the pattern of behaviour at a later stage is said to be predictable from early analysis and observation. The value of early detection in this case has been pointed out by Knobloch & Pasamanick (1960). They have further suggested that:

> The form that behaviour takes as the organism attains maturity can be delineated quite precisely in terms of direction, tempo, inter-relationships and complexity.

In the evaluation of any diagnostic test or study of the behavioural effects of neurological dysfunction the whole question of the relationship between maturational level and chronological age demands a careful consideration. The difficulty of differentiating between developmental retardation and actual (minimal) brain damage can only be resolved in the light of these considerations.

This problem was appreciated by Gesell & Amatruda (1941). They realised the possibility that children with organic brain damage could be diagnosed in the first few months of life on the basis of a disturbance in motor and adaptive development. They acknowledged that functional tests of behaviour did not differentiate between the level of maturity and the efficiency of the Central Nervous System. With diagnostic tests dealing with movements involving hand-eye coordination, Gesell (1941) attempted to alleviate the influence of maturational level. Unlike other tests of neural dysfunction all the items that were used involved coordinated actions that were the result

of specific practice and therefore not acquired through maturation. From this behavioural approach the Gesell Developmental
and Neurological Examination procedure was formulated.
This later proved to be a valid and reliable means of identifying
abnormalities in distinctive behavioural patterns.

Tests of motor impairment

Since the effects of brain damage often appear as deficiencies
in motor ability and performance, as in the various conditions
of cerebral palsy, many of the earlier tests that have been used
in a diagnosis of motor impairment have been tests of brain
damage. The results of studies of children with visuo-motor
disturbances and associated learning problems have revealed
substantial evidence of defects and developmental retardation
in perceptual and other functions of mental activity. Although
acknowledging the vast amount of work that has been done in
attempting to reveal the organic origin of such defects, it is felt
that this approach is of little value to the educationalist.

In answer to the preceding observations there is evidence to
suggest that the following procedures may be of value not only
in diagnosing the root cause of impairment but also in identifying some of the difficulties that restrict *present* learning.

For the purposes of convenience, this information has been
grouped under four main headings, and arranged in the
order in which it is most likely to be gathered.

1. Teachers' and/or parents' assessment.
   (*a*) Observation of motor performances.
   (*b*) Information from school and other records,
      (i) educational background (e.g. reading and arith-
          metic abilities),
      (ii) intelligence tests,
      (iii) medical history,
      (iv) home background.
2. Medical examinations.
   (*a*) Physical and neurological examinations involving
        the testing of sight, hearing, etc.: reflexes, muscle
        coordination and tone, etc.
   (*b*) Electroencephalograph examination.
   (*c*) Motor impersistence tests.
3. Motor proficiency tests that have been specifically designed
   to assist in the diagnosis of some of the conditions of motor
   impairment.

(*a*) The Oseretzky tests (1923, 1931).
(*b*) Yarmolenko's test (1933).
(*c*) The Lincoln/Oseretzky Revision (Sloan, 1953).
(*d*) The Vineland Adaption of the Oseretzky tests (Cassell, 1949).
(*e*) A general test of Motor Impairment (Stott, 1966).

The evolution of these tests represents a noticeable shift of attention away from the traditional concept that has associated motor disabilities with brain damage. The traditional view has, however, persisted and still dominates the approach to the subject. This may be accounted for by the fact that the use of these tests has been largely restricted to the severe cases of motor disability where the symptoms of brain damage are more obvious.

It is unfortunate that this association has been so firmly established for it has diverted attention away from the exploration of other lines of approach. The possibility that the neural factor in many of the cases of motor impairment may stem from circumstances other than those of brain damage has remained relatively unexplored. As a result of this situation a child with obvious difficulties in skill learning may not be recognised as being impaired because of the failure of any test of brain damage to identify the cause.

4. Psychometric tests designed to detect deficiencies (in maturational abilities) that appear to be at least partly responsible for certain difficulties in motor skills learning and performance.

    (i) Tests used to identify brain damage:
        e.g. (*a*) The Bender Gestalt test (1938)
        (*b*) The Memory for Designs test (Graham & Kendall, 1960).
    (ii) Tests of sophistication of body-concept:
        e.g. (*a*) Draw-a-man test (Witkin, 1966).
    (iii) Tests of specific factors of motor performance:
    (*a*) Manual dexterity, e.g. the Minnesota rate of manipulation test.
    (*b*) Psycho-motor test of speed and accuracy, e.g. Spiral Maze test (Gibson, 1964).
    (iv) Tests of intelligence: e.g. the Wechsler Intelligence Scale for Children (1949).
    (v) Tests of perceptual abilities:
        e.g. Developmental Test of Visual Perception (Frostig, 1963).

Discussion of the sources of diagnostic information
Under this heading the discussion has been confined to those tests with which parents and educationalists are perhaps least familiar.

1. Motor impersistence tests

The recognition of common signs and symptoms may be an important consideration in any medical diagnosis of neural dysfunction. This is facilitated when the signs are clearly defined and relatively unambiguous. In this respect studies of the behaviour of children whose perceptual-motor disabilities are caused by brain damage have revealed certain characteristic tendencies which indicate learning difficulties.

Many of these children have shown disturbances in perception, concept formation, and emotional behaviour, either separately or in combination. The perceptive and conceptual deviations have been associated with such behavioural characteristics as distractibility, short attention span, perseveration, and disinhibition, together with disturbances in visual, auditory, and tactile perception.

Kolburne (1965) has referred to this behaviour as a syndrome characteristic of children with minimal brain damage. Even though the neurological signs of brain injury were not seen to be present, and the electroencephalogram tracings often negative, he reported that:

> nearly all the mildly brain injured children have most of these characteristics to a greater or lesser degree.

In one of the more easily recognisable forms of this behaviour it has frequently been observed that even the mild cases of brain damage are seemingly incapable of maintaining certain voluntary acts for any length of time.

As early as 1907, Lewandowsky felt that the inability to maintain the eyes closed as an apractic disorder. In 1924 Pineas noticed patients with hemiplegia also showed an 'inability to keep the eyes closed'. A similar observation was made by Zutt in 1950. He added the characteristic of the inability to 'keep the tongue protruded'.

In the following year Fisher (1956) proposed the term 'Motor Impersistence' and identified the following characteristics, all of which were almost exclusively associated with damage to the non-dominant hemisphere:

1. Inability to maintain gaze in any one direction ('ocular vacillation'), or to keep eyes fixed centrally under the distraction of the examiner's finger movements ('attraction response').
2. Inability to keep mouth open and/or tongue protruded.
3. Difficulty in keeping eyelids shut during sensory testing.
4. Difficulty in making a prolonged 'ah' sound.
5. Difficulty in exerting steady pressure during hand gripping.

The presence of defects in motor performances and in sensory perception were also noted.

Following these reports, a systematic clinical investigation was carried out with 101 brain damaged patients and a matched control group by Joynt, Benton & Fogel (1962). Using a battery of nine tests, with a time scoring system, they found that 23% of the brain damaged group showed pathological impersistence. They also concluded that motor impersistence of a pathological degree was associated with such factors as mental impersistence and disorientation of place, person and time.

This view was also taken by Rutter, Graham & Birch (1966) in a detailed analysis of these factors. They observed that motor impersistence, as indicated by choreiform movements, was more closely related to mental age than to any specific educational disability.

Prechtl & Stemmer (1962) used similar tests with the objective of searching for the aetiological factors in the behaviour of certain problem children who had been referred to the doctor because of poor school ability and as showing signs of excessive activity and restlessness. These hyperkinetic symptoms ranged from a slight lack of physical skill to the more serious disturbance of the pyramidal system. The investigation was carried out with a group of fifty children aged between 9 and 12 years. In describing their behaviour, Prechtl & Stemmer state:

The movements were slight and jerky and occur quite irregularly arythmically in different muscles. They are characterised by sudden occurrence and short duration. Muscles of the tongue, face, neck and trunk were involved in all of these cases. . . . A disturbance in coordination (finger-nose; heel-toe tests) depended on the intensity of choreiform twitches but this was also due to Dyskinesia and not to a true ataxia.

In consideration of the aetiology, they believed that this choreiform syndrome was the result of injury to the infant's nervous system by 'pre-, para- or postnatal complications', as shown by the case histories.

Garfield (1964) in a study with twenty-five brain damaged children, aged between 5 and 11 years, and twenty-five normal children, matched for age, sex and intelligence, found that on six of the eight tasks the brain damaged children were significantly poorer than the controls ($P < 0.05$). In discussing the significance of this phenomenon and the value of such tests as a useful means of clinical diagnosis, he observed:

> The utilisation of these tests must enable one to identify the brain damaged child without gross motor impairment and to differentiate the child whose behaviour difficulties are a function of Central Nervous System impairment (i.e. neurological dysfunction) from the child with psychogenic behaviour problems.

In a later study with Benton & MacQueen (1966), Garfield paired twenty-two cultural familial retardates with twenty-two brain damaged children and tested them on the eight tasks used previously by Fisher. The study was designed to investigate the hypothesis that these retardates who were pathologically impersistent showed evidence of brain damage. The superiority of the former group on all eight tests was striking, and performance of a large number of the brain damaged children was far from perfect. The incidence of motor impersistence in both groups was found to be independent of IQ, although it was noted with conviction that physical immaturity, or the lack of it, was an important factor. The results showed that a high screening efficiency (93%) was obtained by the use of these tests.

A recent study of the phenomena of motor impersistence was conducted as part of a more general survey by Yule, Graham & Tizard (1967) with a group of 2,200 children aged between 9 and 10 years, who were resident in the Isle of Wight. From this number 450 children were selected on the basis of poor performance on educational tests, and 159 normal children were added, making a group of approximately 600 who were investigated more intensively. The motor impersistence tests involved seven commonly accepted standard tasks.

From their observations it was seen that dyspraxic and choreiform movements were both associated with motor impersistence, and there was also evidence of a correlation between motor impersistence and psychiatric disorders. Their conclusions regarding the relationship of motor impersistence and clumsiness are particularly significant:

> There is evidence, however, of the specificity of impersistence in the area of motor skills. Clumsy children in the Yule, Graham and Tizard research had impaired motor coordination and a high degree of motor impersistence even when the lower than average IQ was taken into account. Definite evidence has been produced showing the close link between brain damage and motor impersistence.

Studies such as these provide a valuable background of information regarding the characteristics of certain forms of motor impairment caused by neural dysfunction. Any effective diagnostic test must surely be based on a consideration of these observed and known characteristics.

2. Motor proficiency tests that have been specifically designed to assist in the diagnosis of some of the conditions of motor impairment.

The Oseretzky tests

Previous work in the field of diagnostic tests of motor impairment has been very limited. The most relevant and detailed study of the subject was initiated by the Russian Oseretzky, and subsequent developments appear very much related to his original work as part of a chain of progressive research and development of the subject.

The Oseretzky tests, first published in 1923, from the Psychoneurological Clinic in Moscow, were designed to aid in a very broad diagnosis of neurological and motor deficiency. The initial research was prompted by clinical observations of children of apparently normal or above IQ, who showed striking deficiency in motor performance up to a point which was described as 'motor idiocy'. Oseretzky believed that such deficiency could have marked social and/or clinical implications.

It is conceivable that a child could be making poor adjustment from a social and personality point of view because of 'motor awkwardness'.

His test was intended to be a useful measure of the severity of this 'awkwardness', in order to assist the teacher in developing an effective remedial programme to help the child improve his physical performance.

The initial standardisation of his Motor Development Scale of 1923 consisted only of 410 children (195 boys and 215 girls) with the exclusion of children with somatic or neurological defects. In 1925, however, a further attempt to standardise the items of his test was made with a control group of 1,500 normal and 200 psychotic, nervous and psychopathic children.

Attempts were then made to calculate the 'motor age' of a child on the same principle as the Binet Scale for Intelligence. From the results of a child's performance at successive age levels his grade of motor deficiency was calculated, on the following basis:

Light $1-1\frac{1}{2}$ years below chronological age.
Medium $1\frac{1}{2}-3$ years below chronological age.
Great 3–5 years below chronological age.
Idiocy below 5 years below chronological age.

It appears that the scale was later modified and proved of value in the examination of adults, by providing the means for assessing the relationship between motor ability, character, and somatic constitution (according to Kretschner's Somatic Type). This information was used in vocational guidance.

Five basic factors, or 'motor components', were contained in the original Metric Scale. Additional items were later added in order to extend the range of the tests further to assist in determining the appropriate educational assignments for clinical cases of motor deficiency.

To the following list of original items have been added Vandenberg's assessment (1964) of the origin of their innervation and control.

1. MOTOR SPEED,
   'a complex combination of tempo (under the control of striate mechanisms and activated by frontal thalamic system), the innervation—denervation cycle (stryo-cerebellar system) and the degree of development of automatised motor responses (localised in the cortex). All these are under some control of the higher cortical centres'.
2. SIMULTANEOUS VOLUNTARY MOVEMENTS (with precision of movements),
   'dependent on the highest motoric cortical centres'.
3. STATIC COORDINATION (associated with static balance),
   'it presumes the intactness of the cerebellar systems and the vestibular and other sensory appreciation connected with the cerebellum'.
4. DYNAMIC COORDINATION. (This later included manual dexterity.)
5. GENERAL COORDINATION.
   Both this and the item of dynamic coordination are concerned with balance and control of the body in movement.
   Gurewitch, the director of the Psychoneurological Clinic in Moscow, considered this component to be under the control of all motoric systems of the brain but particularly of the frontal cerebellar mechanisms.
6. SYNKINESIA (surplus associated movements), 'dependent on the highest motoric cortical centres'.

In order to extend the range of the test the following items were later added.

7. Rhythmic ability.*
8. Motor strength.*
9. Formulation of motor formulas.
10. Speed of mental set.
11. Automatised motor action.
12. Orientation in space.
13. Regulation of innervation and denervation.
14. Automatic defence reactions.

From further studies with children aged between 4 and 14 years, it was observed that the motor performance of boys and girls were alike up to the age of 8 years. After that two

*These items were found to be unsuitable for successive year-by-year grading in the Metric Scale since few reliable tests of them were devised, and others required complex apparatus.

L

different scales were found to be necessary in order to accommodate the varying types of performance. This assumption was
based upon the impressions of the investigators who were asked
to make descriptive notes during the subject's performance.
They observed that girls were quicker and more rhythmic
and boys stronger and more coordinated in the voluntary
simultaneous movements.

It was also observed that no relationship existed between
motor and mental development as measured by the Terman
tests, in children of average or above intelligence. With children
known to be mentally retarded, however, a correlation of
0·7 between Motor and Intelligence Quotients was computed,
although it was noted that the tests may not have been appropriate for the more severe cases. This difficulty is explained in
Lassner's (1964) reference:

> True motor retardation had to be distinguished from the
> physical impossibility of executing a task as a consequence of
> a pathological state of the muscular system, or of bodily
> deformation.

Similar difficulties were encountered several years later
(1934 and 1935) when Oseretzky and Payova used the test
to investigate the motor capacity of children with known defects
and diseases which included cases of poliomyelitis and defective
peripheral appreciation. Their results appeared to be sufficiently
informative as to enable them to draw certain conclusions
regarding the pathology of the diseases.

In spite of the extensive use of the Oseretzky Scale in nine
European countries, none of the publications previously referred
to are reported to have included sufficient data or experimental evidence to satisfy any great claims of reliability and
validity.

A revival of the test was made in 1966 by Yule and others
from the Department of Child Development at London
University. They used a shortened form of twelve selective
items in a study of 2,200 children on the Isle of Wight. The items
selected required the minimum of equipment and were
arranged in order of difficulty to discriminate within the age
range of 9–10 years. It was intended to investigate the hypothesis that 'motor clumsiness is associated with educationally
handicapping conditions'. The items were reported to be 'a

mixture involving gross motor control (e.g. balance on one leg) and fine motor coordination (e.g. picking up match sticks)'. Using the scoring system that allowed two trials for each test (3 points were given for pass on first trial, 2 points on second trial, 1 point for doubtful pass on second trial, and no score for complete failure) the maximum possible raw score was 57 points (including separate scores for each hand or foot on seven of the items).

FINDINGS:

1. In a test-retest study of reliability from 1–29 days (Mean = 7·8 days) a correlation of 0·69 was computed. This was reported to be almost as high as that found by Sloan after one year.

2. In an analysis of validity, Yule reported:

Of all the correlations between raw scores and a wide variety of IQ and attainment measures in the control group, only age correlated significantly at the 1% level ($r = 0·31$).

3. In relation to IQ, in the control group of normal children, the correlations between the Oseretzky score and that of the W.I.S.C. test was – 0·002.

4. Correlations between each individual item and the total raw score ranged from 0·24 to 0·57, all were found to be statistically significant ($P < 0·001$).

Using the raw score an assumed identification of clumsiness was made on the following basis,

Severely clumsy   = 2σ or below appropriate age level mean score.
Moderately clumsy   = Between 1σ and 2σ below.
Normal   = Upwards from 1σ below mean.

5. From the group of neurologically handicapped children a strong relationship was found between IQ and severe clumsiness. This was accentuated in the lower levels of IQ. The severely clumsy children were therefore found to be more retarded both intellectually and educationally (their mean IQ score on W.I.S.C. was equivalent to a standardised score of 83).

In conclusion it was reported that,

Motor clumsiness may take its place with those other

developmental disabilities such as adverse reading retardation, hyperkinesis, or developmental speech disorders in which a clear association with age and IQ is linked to an inconsistent but none the less definite association with brain damage Yule (1967).

Van der Lugt, a Dutch psychologist, used the tests in 1939 and revised the psychomotor profile to give a metric study of manual ability. This revision, although used in several French-speaking countries, was not translated into English until twenty years later.

From her experience of the Oseretzky test she made certain observations and criticisms both of the content and technique of administration. She recorded that the individual tests appeared to have been selected somewhat indiscriminately as regards both their diagnostic significance and any allowance for sex differences. In addition to the complicated and lengthy administrative procedure caused by the large number of tests and rather vague instructions, she observed that performances on some of the items were almost certainly influenced by the practice opportunities afforded by certain environments.

Similar shortcomings of the test were expressed by Yarmolenko (1933), a colleague of Oseretzky and an important figure in the Russian movement.

It is not enough to say that a child's motor co-efficient is normal for his chronological age, or that he surpasses it. The data must be analysed.

She found the diagnostic possibilities inadequate for her research and so devised her own motor scale based on the more fundamental elements of 'life essential movements' such as walking and grasping, etc. This she standardised on schoolchildren aged between 8 and 15 years. This revision also included motor profiles from which a child was regarded as normal if all points were contained between plus and minus 1σ.

She appears to have also criticised the basic assumption made by Oseretzky that each of his first seven items or components represented various 'motor systems'. In his diagnostic procedure the effective functioning of each system was roughly appraised from a similar motor profile obtained from each child's performance. The profile was therefore seen to indicate specific strength or weakness in the areas or 'systems' of motor competency.

It must be noted at this point that these areas were not empirically defined, and a factor analysis (Vandenburg, 1964) has since failed to establish their independence. The profile measured the deviation of each of the various components above and below the mean performance.

Oseretzky had admitted that discrepancies existed between the relative diagnostic values of certain items, and some appeared to be associated with skills already acquired. The method of testing he used started the child at his own age level and continued at progresssive levels upwards and down until two successive passes and two successive failures were recorded. The total points scored were then referred to the standardised Metric Scale and related to chronological age to give a 'Motor Quotient' or 'Motorik'.

The number of tests for each item was originally so time-consuming that in a later revision Oseretzky reduced this to five for each of the first six items that were then employed. This provided thirty tests (as opposed to eighty-five in the original) for each age group. The time factor was largely overcome by a new system of group testing. It was claimed that 20–25 subjects (12–15 younger or problem children) could be examined simultaneously in 45 minutes for normal, and 1 hour for abnormal children.

The validity of this method would seem to stand or fall by the accuracy of the standardisation of each item for the different age groups. A child who passed an item at his own age level and failed at the one below would receive an inappropriate score. It is assumed, therefore, that the two successes and failures would appear in correct consecutive order.

The only French translation of the Oseretzky revision of 1931 was published in Belgium in 1934. It included the scoring system and method of calculating the motor age of a child. This prompted some enthusiastic work with the tests at the Mental Hygiene Clinic at Brussels by Decroly & Bratu (1934). Their studies in this field produced definite progress, particularly with the introduction of more efficient teaching methods for the handicapped. Remedial exercises were adapted more suitably to the child's motor capacity and the effects of fatigue in certain functions were studied in more relevant detail.

From this French translation Juarros (1939), working in Spain, revised a number of items of the Oseretzky test in order to achieve a quicker and more accurate measure by group examination. In his battery he replaced the test of synkinesis with an item of motor strength which he called 'Force', and also identified 'Manual Coordination' in terms of tests of precision of movement. His work appears to have been concerned with attempts to determine the motor age and subsequent physical development of children with only minor degrees of motor impairment. In this connection he believed in the practical value of these tests in the physical education programme of normal children from the point of view of identifying the physical characteristics of psychotic and neurotic children.

Previous to the one English translation the only reference in America to the work of Oseretzky came from the studies of Kopp (1943) in Paris and New York, with stuttering children. It is interesting to note that, using the Oseretzky test taken from the French translation in Brussels, she found evidence of marked disturbances in the motor function of these children and formed the opinion that stuttering was more of a neurological than psychological disorder. She reported that:

> Even in cases not exhibiting motor retardation, analysis of their scores revealed uniform deficiency in the maturity of the extrapyramidal system, shown by failure in the tests for synkinesis, mimicry, rhythm, and coordination.

Of these functions she observed the greatest deficiency in the items dealing with synkinetic movements and static coordination. Using Oseretzky's four broad categories of motor deficiency (mentioned earlier) she found that 46% of the stuttering children tested came under the category of 'Motor Idiots', and an additional 46% recorded failures in items at more than one year below their age level. She concluded that the motor deficiency was part of the same condition responsible for this and possibly other related speech disorders.

The most significant English translation of the Oseretzky Scale was sponsored and edited by Doll at the Vineland Laboratory in America in 1946. The translation was made by Fosa from da Costa's Portuguese version published in 1943. Writing at the time of the translation, Doll (1946) stated:

The use of this scale will materially facilitate a better under-standing of the limitations of mentally deficient children and adults in respect to motor coordination and the practical aspects of motor proficiency.

In his editorial review, Doll (1946) made reference to the value of the tests in the educational field.

The educator will need to know the value of the child's motor reactions and their causes, so that he may try to train to control and coordinate his movements, improving with selected exercise those which are most deficient in order that the child may acquire manual ability, skill, and motor equilibrium. It is in this field that the Oseretzky tests can provide him with an excellent gauge.

The Lincoln/Oseretzky test

In 1948 and again in 1953 and 1955, following the Vineland translation, Sloan (1955) published the Lincoln Adaption of the Oseretzky tests from Lincoln State School, Illinois.

In the first instance only those items were selected that minimised any cultural or sex bias and permitted reliable scoring. Sloan also disregarded those that required elaborate testing materials and those that were believed to have a signifi-cant positive correlation with age. In all, therefore, only thirty-six of the original eighty-five items were retained.

From this beginning he reviewed the whole administrative structure of the Scale. Attempts were made to arrange the items in order of difficulty and establish at least tentative norms for each age group so that a child's performance could be repre-sented as a percentile rank (in order to convert an otherwise meaningless score into a position on a percentile scale).

An analysis of the results of the proceeding studies showed the homogeneous nature of the test. They revealed split-half relia-bility coefficients of 0·96 for males and 0·97 for females, which indicated a considerable overlap of items measuring the same factor or the same relatively few common factors.

In view of its limited range one can only assume that the test now showed certain limitations as a means of actually identifying the various forms of motor impairment. From the evidence of previous studies in America, it was (and still is) commonly accepted that motor skills are relatively specific and show low inter-correlations, particularly when different parts of the body are involved.

Perrin (1921) in an attempted analysis of 'motor ability' used the following three selected motor tests.

1. Bogardus fatigue test (placing cubes on a cube by rotating arms of a machine).
2. Card sorting into suits into four boxes.
3. Coordination test (tracing triangles using each hand simultaneously).

He also used tests of fourteen 'Elementary Motor Functions' (including reaction time, static and dynamic balance, rhythm, arm and leg strength). The correlation coefficients between these tests were found to be non-significant almost without exception.

He concluded that motor ability was influenced by a number of specific factors acting simultaneously and a 'few general modes of motor reaction', influenced by a general factor related to character and intelligence.

Using similar tests of assumed factors of motor ability (including, aiming, tracing, tapping, manual dexterity—matches into boxes, and simple auditory reaction time), Muscio (1922) found the highest correlation between items to be 0·4, this being the comparison between left and right hand coordination.

In this field also, Seashore (1930), using tests related to the practical (vocational) application of motor skills (hand-eye coordination, speed of hand, bimanual speed and precision), found an average correlation of 0·25 and concluded that there was no common factor of motor ability. Seashore (1928) also reported that Binet, in his work with motor tests and their relationship with motor ability nearly thirty years earlier, had come to very similar conclusions.

This can be viewed as a general point of criticism of all the revisions of the Oseretzky tests at this time. Many seemed prepared to accept the value of these tests as a diagnostic aid in eliciting certain physical traits or characteristic behaviour patterns of children with known neural dysfunction. There is no evidence, however, that motor performance tests of this type were used for the initial diagnosis or identification of impaired function. Then, as today, the mild cases of motor impairment were seen to be an effect rather than a cause of some form of psychological, social, mental or nervous mal-adjustment. In the absence of any assumed causative role, therefore, the need for early diagnosis and treatment was not fully realised.

In the Oseretzky original and in the Lincoln and other revisions, the six items appeared to be more descriptive of activities involved in motor performance than actual components of motor ability. No claims were made that one test measured one factor to the exclusion of any others. Indeed, in a factor analytical study, Thams (1955) found that there were only 342 out of 1,332 items which correlated more than 0·28.

It is believed that the six 'components' of the Oseretzky test were chosen to represent the predominant and most fundamental areas of motor ability. For example, Oseretzky included tests of 'Throwing a ball', and fine finger movements as a measure of one and the same component notably 'Manual coordination', yet the former involves gross hand (arm)-eye coordination whereas the latter was taken by Stott (1966) as a test of manual dexterity.

This apparent discrepancy was observed by Vandenburg (1964) who noted that:

> All the items of the Oseretzky and Lincoln/Oseretzky appear to require the operation of all or most of the six components and are not singly or primarily dependent upon the component they are supposed to measure.

Emphasis was therefore placed in the Lincoln revision upon the Developmental Scale, and maturational and learning factors were apparently allowed to register an important influence on the subject's performance, for the subject's scores increased with age. Using the data from the preliminary sample a correlation of total score with age was computed as 0·87 for males and 0·88 for females. In a sense, therefore, these were regarded as validity coefficients.

Vandenburg, in his analysis of the Lincoln/Oseretzky test, saw the possibilities of the Developmental Scale, not only as a predictor of adolescent athletic ability but also for its clinical value of assisting in the detection of cerebral palsy in children:

> It is conceivable . . . that impaired motor performance is the result of a common precursor, be this a biochemical abnormality or a reduced participation in normal ventures and

adventures in childhood and adolescence. As an alternative it is conceivable that the impaired motor development contributes to mental illness or at least is closer to the true causes of it than are measures of cognitive skills.

He observed that the correlations between the items were generally low, and suggested that the nature of the factors measured by the Oseretzky test needed further clarification.

The Vineland adaption of the Oseretzky tests

In 1949, three years after the English translation of the Oseretzky tests work began on the Vineland Adaption at the training school at Vineland, New Jersey. Scientific research in the measurement of motor aptitudes had been progressing for many years. Here the development of the 'Vineland Maturity Scale' for social competence prompted the desire for a more systematic measurement of motor proficiency from the point of view of maturation and development. The translation was made mainly in order to use the Oseretzky Scale to complete this work.

Research was undertaken in this project by Cassell (1949). His revision followed a study of the comparison of currently approved tests of motor ability, notably the Iowa revision of the Brace tests (McCloy, 1934), the Metheny/Johnson test (Metheny, 1938) and the Cowan/Pratt 'hurdle jump test' (1934) with the Lincoln/Oscretzky revision.

Much of Cassell's work on the Vineland Adaption concentrated more upon simplifying the method of administration of the Oseretzky Scale than on any new concepts of neurological diagnosis. The tasks were selected to provide a more objective scoring system, and based upon this criteria, all tests of synkinesia, known to be difficult to score, were omitted. Although the tests were reported to be a valuable measure capable of discriminating between endogenous and exogenous mental defectives, no standardisation procedure was pursued.

The work was apparently associated with that of Doll, at the Training School Centre, who was concerned with the general problem of aetiology of brain damaged children.

Previously, the most effective measure of the development of motor performance in children, used by the Centre, was believed to be the railwalking test devised by Heath (1953). Although the form of his test appears to be somewhat over-simplified, there is no doubt that his work was held in high regard particularly for his conclusions regarding the psychological implications of the effects of motor disability.

Amongst his findings Heath observed that the conflict that arose as a result of the continual discrepancy between the aspired level and the actual level of the performances of a 'motor defective' not only caused tension but also created an emotional trend that was difficult to control. The modified performance influenced by the natural feedback or 'reflective criticism' was often seen to be slower and even less effective than previous attempts. It was also recorded that attempts to increase the speed of reaction often led to more diffuse and inaccurate movements.

Although the Vineland Adaption was intended to provide a more composite picture than the railwalking test, its application appears to have followed the same restricted usage. Little or no attempt was made to apply the test in the diagnosis of any but the known cases of neural dysfunction.

It was not until 1960 that Gollnitz, a German neuropsychiatrist, for the first time concentrated specifically on the idea of an assessment of impairment as opposed to the ability of brain damaged children. From this point of view, items from the Oseretzky Scale were selected and grouped on the basis that only a very small percentage of children should fail. These were then tested at successive lower levels until all the items were passed. This revision can be seen as a breakaway from the previous tests which attempted to calculate the motor age of a child and to draw conclusions on the basis of comparisons with the performances of normal children. Gollnitz was not concerned with a measure of motor ability nor with the performance of children who passed the test, for under this criteria, success at the basal age level did not indicate the child's motor age.

A general test of motor impairment for children

In 1966 Stott et al. produced a test of motor impairment based on Gollnitz's revision of the Oseretzky test. His main criteria for item choice was that motor disability should be reasonably attributed to neural dysfunction. This he said could be inferred if there is a failure to control or coordinate simple actions without discernable physical disability. The inference becomes more of a probability if the incompetence is observed in diverse functions. He also acknowledged the difficulty of minimising the effect of other irrelevant factors present in all such empirical tests:

> Since behaviour involves the whole person it can be affected by incompetence in any of a number of functions—perceptual, intellectual, motivational (emotional) or muscular . . . it is a question of reducing their influence on the result by choosing activities which are relatively non-discriminating in these areas.

Differences in previous learning, in cultural environments, and in educational opportunity were also seen to present problems of item choice that could not be completely eliminated. Both familiarity with the activity and a knowledge of the physical properties of any object that is manipulated, are relevant factors of the experience necessary in the accomplishment of any set task. Such experience will differ with each subject, whether it is from either previous practice, of throwing for example, or familiarity with a tennis ball. The danger of selecting items that are more free from cultural familiarity is that they may become divorced from the fundamental activities of real life.

With these considerations in mind, Stott selected five tasks for each level from 5 to 14 years, as a test of the first five of Oseretzky's original items ('dynamic manual coordination' was modified to 'manual dexterity'). The sixth item, 'synkinesis', was measured by three standard tests for all ages at the beginning of the test proceedings. In view of the understanding that neural dysfunction can be specific to one function or one part of the body, the six items were thought to be suitable in as much as they showed a reasonably comprehensive sampling of motor activity. Whether they represent the essential factors of motor performance sufficiently accurately to provide a means of detecting impairment, is still very much open to question.

It was Stott's intention that the test should be applied in schools in conjunction with the teachers' assessment as an initial screening device.

In a study by Whiting et al. (1969) the effectiveness of Stott's test as a screening device was investigated in both a clinical and a child guidance setting.

In a clinical situation, 108 children who were attending a paediatric out-patient clinic were tested. These children whose ages ranged from 4 to 16 years, were being examined or receiving treatment for any of a complete range of disorders.

The validation took the form of a comparison of a child's performance on Stott's test with a paediatrician's diagnosis and assessment of his case. The results, as indicated in the table below, showed that of the five children who were diagnosed by Stott's test as being impaired, only one was not confirmed by the clinical diagnosis. In addition, however, there were three clinically diagnosed cases of motor impairment that were not screened off by the test.

TABLE 8

Screening efficiency of Stott test and clinical diagnoses: out-patient population

| Test diagnosis | Paediatric diagnosis | | Totals |
	Not impaired	Impaired	
Not impaired	98	3	101
Impaired	1	4	5
Totals	99	7	106

$$\chi^2 = 5\cdot95; \ P < 0\cdot02$$

In the child guidance centre, ten children who were receiving remedial teaching were selected for testing because they had been noticed by either their parents, teachers or examining psychologists as being 'clumsy or having some form of motor disorganisation'. By their performance on Stott's test, only four of these ten children were identified as being impaired.

TABLE 9

Screening efficiency of Stott test and diagnoses of parent, teacher or psychologist: child guidance population

	Not impaired	Impaired	Totals
Diagnosis of parent, teacher or psychologist	0	10	10
Stott Test	6	4	10
Totals	6	14	20

$$\chi^2 = 8\cdot56; \ P < 0\cdot01$$

It was also recorded that a paediatrician's examination of these four children revealed 'no significant abnormalities'. On the basis of these results, the validity of the test as a screening device is at least questionable.

A further attempt was made by Whiting *et al.* (1969) to validate Stott's test by comparing its screening efficiency with that of the teacher's subjective assessment.

In reply to a questionnaire, teachers in twenty-two schools submitted the names of fifty children aged 8 years, whom they regarded as being clumsy. The criteria for this assessment included that of 'an inability or a poor standard of performance in one of a combination of simple physical skills'. From their performance on Stott's test only thirteen of these showed any real evidence to support this claim.

It seemed apparent that the considerable discrepancy here may have been due to the clouding effect that disorders in the general behaviour of some of the children may have had on the teachers' assessment of their capabilities. This does not deny the possibility that a child's inability may be either a causative or consequential factor in his general conduct and attitude to schoolwork. The fact that ten of the fifty children passed all items at their own age level may have demonstrated that these particular subtests are not sufficiently sensitive to the more mild cases of impairment. This would imply that the children who were differentiated were those with the most severe impairment.

From these results it was also interesting to note that the childrens' scores on items 1, 2 and 4 (static balance, hand-eye coordination, and manual dexterity) compared very closely to their scores on all five items of the test (correlation coefficient of 0·95). This suggests that a score based on these three subtests of Stott's test might be as efficient a screening device as that of the complete set of five subtests. It may also point to a possible weakness of the test reflected in an overlapping of the factors to an extent which would make some subtests redundant. An item-analysis would no doubt shed some light on this issue.

3. *Psychometric tests* designed to detect deficiencies (in maturational abilities) that appear to be at least partly responsible for certain difficulties in motor skills learning and performance.

In this section there appears only a sample of the many

tests that have been used with varying degrees of success in the diagnosis of these deficiencies. The choice has been made in order to represent some of the common and more significant lines of approach. The contributions of these have proved to be extremely valuable to their own areas of inquiry, while others appear to have equally relevant possibilities.

(i) *Tests used to identify brain damage*

The major weakness of tests of brain damage has been the absence of an adequate theory of brain function upon which they can be based. It has been a common practice among those engaged in the validation of these tests to make a classification of 'brain damage' versus 'non-brain damage'. Even so, the overlap of scores between these two groups may be considerable, despite the statistically significant difference between the group means. Not only has this differentiation by psychological tests been frequently conducted with fairly clear-cut criterion groups, but the implication is that the research has been concerned simply with the question of the presence or absence of injury.

Assuming that such a differentiation was reliable how much would this contribute to the task of making a diagnosis? The value of diagnosis in this context lies in its descriptive functions and its implications of prognosis and treatment rather than of aetiology (if these aspects can, in fact, be separated). A label of 'brain damaged' is of little use in dealing with the main problem of compensatory education. This unqualified use of the term is a gross over-simplification of all that is involved. There is considerable evidence of many behavioural abnormalities and types of deficit produced by brain injuries. The identification of a child suffering from some learning disability or perceptual abnormality would be much more useful than the label 'brain damaged'. Cruickshank *et al.* (1961) have suggested that neurological diagnosis in itself can rarely be translated into a dynamic educational programme. It would be extremely narrow and short-sighted if future investigations into the causes of impairment were limited to this unitary criteria of brain damage.

(a) The Bender-Gestalt test

Many well-known techniques such as the Bender-Gestalt,

the Graham-Kendall Memory for designs test or Benton Visual Retention test, predict the presence or absence of brain damage no better than some other procedures not published in test form, e.g. word fluency or right-left discrimination. This suggests that, at the present time, screening devices should be selected on the basis of sound test construction and validation procedures rather than minimal differences in hit rate derived from the few available studies.

Spreen & Benton (1965)

The Bender-Gestalt test was originally devised in 1938 for children over the age of 4 years. Later modifications by Hutt & Briskin (1960) and Clawson (1962) have adapted the test for children within more specific age ranges. At the present time the most widely used version has come from the work of Koppitz (1964) who revised the scoring technique of Pascal & Suttell (1951) and produced the Developmental Bender Scoring System for children aged between 4 and 12 years.

The test consists of eight designs which are copied by the child under standardised conditions. The scoring system identifies a total of thirty errors which may or may not be present in the child's drawings. These errors have been standardised against performances of 195 first and second grade children on the Metropolitan Achievement test (Hildreth & Griffiths, 1946). An example of the reliability of scoring has been provided by Miller et al. (1963) who achieved statistically significant correlations ranging between 0·88 and 0·96 using a Pearson product-moment on thirty sets of original drawings. The consistency of the test scores was investigated on a test–re-test basis after an interval of 4 months, and revealed a rank order correlation of approximately 0·6 (P<0·001). Normative data for the Koppitz scoring system was obtained from the results of over 1,000 children between the ages of 5 and 10 years. The mean scores for the different age groups showed an expected distribution along the developmental scale with no statistically significant differences between the scores of boys and girls at any age level.

Using the test in conjunction with the Metropolitan Achievement test, Koppitz found a significant correlation in respect of the achievements of 7- and 8-year-old children in reading and arithmetic. The common factors suggested to account for this were the importance of 'attention to detail', and the ability to perceive and integrate the parts (i.e. the parts of a design, and the letters of a word) into the whole.

There appears to be some evidence here that the test may be useful in diagnosing the aetiology of a child's reading difficulties either in respect of a retardation in maturation or of more specific problems in visual perception. Claims have also been made of a relationship between the developmental score and the number of emotional indicators on the Bender test but there appears to be little substantive evidence to support these.

A check on the validity of the Koppitz scoring system as a predictor of a child's future reading problems was made by Thweatt (1963) using sixty-one children who were tested initially whilst in their first grade at a public school. It was hypothesised that those who scored *above* the Bender mean composite score for that age group would experience reading problems to some degree. After a lapse of approximately 2 years the same children were examined on the reading vocabulary and reading comprehension subtests of the Durrell Analysis of Reading Difficulty tests. For the purposes of this study they were regarded as having a reading problem if their performances on either or both of the subtests were 5 months or more below their grade placement. The results showed that of the twenty-two children who had scored above the group's Bender mean, fifteen were experiencing reading problems, and as was also predicted *none* of the remaining thirty-nine who had scored on or *below* the group's Bender mean had reading difficulties. In his summary, Thweatt reported:

> The results indicate that the Bender-Gestalt Test with Koppitz's scoring system can predict with accuracy future reading problem cases regardless of the causal factors of the reading disability.

Apart from the support of this and other studies, the popularity of the test must be largely attributed to its simplicity, ease of administration and the intriguing way in which it is scored. No doubt the future possibilities of the test will very much depend upon the progress that is made with the interpretation of the errors in a child's drawings. This would appear to be the approach to a clearer understanding of the nature of a child's difficulties in visual-motor performances,

M

rather more so than a comparative evaluation of the standard of performance.

(b) Memory for Designs test

This test involves the presentation of simple geometric designs and the reproduction of these from immediate memory.

As early as 1920, Foster associated this exercise with the identification of 'organic' impairment, although there appears to be no evidence of a validated test of this type in use at that time. In 1940, an attempt was made by Wood & Shulman to standardise and formulate a reliable scoring system for the Ellis Visual Designs test devised in 1927. Their modifications included the addition of more figures to the original designs in order to provide for a more discriminating range of scores, and a rearrangement of the designs for presentation in order of difficulty.

The recommendation that the stimuli should be of an abstract form, to eliminate the inconsistencies involved in reproducing those that had meaningful associations, was later acknowledged by Graham & Kendall (1947). From their original battery of forty designs they produced a selection of fifteen that were found to be the most promising in terms of the reliability of scoring, and more valid in their discrimination of brain damaged subjects. For example, heavy penalties were incurred against orientation errors and the closing of open figures, both of which were found to be characteristic features of the reproductions by the brain damaged subjects. The score for each response was therefore determined by the number and type of errors made so that a poor performance was represented by a high score.

In their attempted validation of the test, Graham & Kendall (1946) reported a study involving seventy brain damaged subjects and an equal number of controls. Their findings revealed a difference of approximately 8 points between the mean scores of the two groups in favour of the b–d group (control group mean score of 3·47, SD of 4·62, and b–d group mean score of 11·54, SD of 7·3). Both the difference between the two means, and the variances were significant at the 0·01 level. A further analysis revealed that 50% of the b–d group (compared to 4% of the controls) appeared in the so-called 'critical' area of high scores, whilst 21% of the b–d group, and

79% of the controls were found in the 'normal' area with scores below 5.

A cross-validation conducted at a later date revealed a very similar distribution of scores within these areas, and an investigation by Garrett, Price & Deabler (1957) placed more than 67% of the b–d group in the critical area, whilst none of their controls reached this level.

With the possibility that brain damage, even at a minimal level, may be a causative factor in some cases of motor impairment, the evidence from these and other studies indicates that a test such as the Memory for Designs should not be overlooked in any detailed diagnostic investigation of the problem.

For this reason the test was used, along with several others, by Clarke *et al.* (1968) in an attempt to identify children who were motor impaired, from a sample of fifty children at an E.S.N. school and fifty controls at an ordinary primary school. In the past the use of this test had been almost entirely confined to work that involved little more than the confirmation of an organic factor in groups with known brain damage in a straight comparison with groups who had no history of such impairment. One of the main purposes of this study was therefore to examine the ability of this measure to discriminate at the marginal levels of neural dysfunction. Unfortunately, in this situation the screening efficiency of the test could only be assessed by comparison with the findings of other tests. In spite of this the results revealed a remarkably close comparison of scores with those of the brain damaged subjects examined by Graham & Kendall.

Using the same scoring system the E.S.N. group (i.e. children with IQ below 85, mean 68 and SD 7·2) scored as follows (the results of the Graham & Kendall study are bracketed alongside).

Normals   26% (21%)
Borderline 30% (29%)
Critical   44% (50%)

Results of the control group (i.e. children in ordinary primary schools):

Normals   60% (79%)
Borderline 36% (17%)
Critical   4% (4%)

It is interesting to note that in the control group, the teachers' questionnaires indicated that only two children were regarded as being 'clumsy', and it was these who were the only two to be classified as critical on the M.F.D. test.

A pointer to the validity of the test in terms of its sensitivity to differentiate between children who may have a minimal degree of brain damage was indicated by a significantly high correlation ($0 \cdot 75$) with the scores of the E.S.N. group on Stott's test. It is, of course, more than a possibility that the common factor of low IQ was in some way responsible for the low scores on both tests. This observation was partly supported by the presence of a somewhat lower correlation ($0 \cdot 34$) between the scores of the control group (mean IQ $100 \cdot 5$) on both tests.

The possibility of a relationship between neural dysfunction and low intelligence is, however, of little significance here, neither is it relevant to the present discussion to suggest that the former is in any way responsible for the latter. What is important is the effect that low intelligence may have had upon each of the various abilities required for successful performance on this type of test. The fact that the children of low IQ did not successfully reproduce certain designs may have been due to a number of relatively independent factors. Not only were the children expected to understand the nature of the task, but they were also required to be capable of perceiving the figures correctly, of remembering them and of the complex processes of innovating and coordinating the appropriate muscular responses. In such a test there is a tendency to assume that these abilities are all present and functioning correctly. In reality, however, a poor performance on the test may well reflect a child's weakness in any of these functions, and serve as an indication to the investigator of the possibility that this measure is unsuitable for the child. In the strictest sense, therefore, this 'readiness ability' should be independent of the responses that a child actually produces as part of the test. In the laboratory situation steps are normally taken to minimise the influence of these extraneous factors in order to obtain a true measure of the factor under consideration, namely the presence of minimal brain damage.

(ii) *Test of sophistication of body-concept*

Draw-a-man test (Witkin, 1966)

> It is to be recalled that the body image is the most complete Gestalt experience involving the integration of all sensory experience impinging on the organism: it is genetically determined and passes through maturational stages which in the child can be followed through the human drawing.
>
> Bender (1938)

The test was intended to indicate the systematic impression that an individual has of his body, cognitive and effective, conscious and unconscious, formed as a continuing process throughout his growth and development. It involves the child in drawing a human figure on one side of a sheet of paper, and the drawing of a figure of the opposite sex on the other side.

This exercise was originally used by Goodenough (1926) as a measure of intelligence. The scoring system was later revised by Harris (1963) who emphasised the developmental aspect by regarding the drawings as a measure of intellectual maturity. A more specific interpretation was put forward by Machover (1949) who viewed the drawings as an individual's reflection of himself, with his characteristic posture and expressive movements. He emphasised this view even further:

> The figure drawn is related intimately to the impulses, anxieties, conflicts and compensation characteristics of that individual. In some sense, the figure drawn is the person and the paper corresponds to the environment.

The view taken by Machover, that an individual projects his whole personality into his drawings is expressed by reference to 'body concept' in terms of 'body esteem'. Thus his scoring scale acknowledges the personal aspirations of the individual and tends to neglect his 'body awareness'.

Almost the reverse of this appeared in the test developed by Witkin *et al.* (1962) which although based on the original Goodenough scale, aimed at a more specific measure of a person's concept of his body. From a detailed analysis of the drawings they identified three categories of characteristic features:

> (i) Form level of drawing (e.g. shapes of limbs, relative sizes and parts, etc.)

(ii) Identity and sex differentiation (e.g. appropriate features and clothing).

(iii) Level of detailing (e.g. facial expression, presence of neck, eyebrows, etc.

Depending upon the degree and manner in which these are represented, drawings are assessed on the following 5 point scale according to the level of sophistication.

(i)   Most sophisticated.
(ii) Moderately sophisticated.
(iii) Intermediate level of sophistication.
(iv) Moderately primitive.
(v)   Most primitive.

Since there is a possibility that a child who has suffered limitations in movement experience has, as a result, a relatively poor body concept, then a measure of his present level of body awareness would appear to be of value.

On this reasoning the test was selected by Whiting *et al.* (1968) as one of a battery used to identify deficiencies in the skilled performances of 100 children, aged 10 years from an E.S.N. and a primary school.

A sufficient standard of reliability in scoring was achieved with correlations of 0·91 and 0·87 between the rating of two assessors. The findings revealed that from the drawings of the fifty children in the primary school, nine were rated at the 'most sophisticated' level and none appeared in the 'most primitive' category. From the E.S.N. group, however, no child scored at the highest level, while twenty-three produced drawings that were regarded as 'most primitive'. One noticeable feature of the correlation matrix for the test battery was the absence of a significant relationship between the scores of the E.S.N. group on this test and the Embedded Figures test (Witkin (1950). There may well have been other factors, perhaps associated with low intelligence, that were equally responsible for the poor drawings of these children.

(iii) *Tests of specific factors of motor performance*

(*a*) Manual dexterity—The Minnesota rate of manipulation test (M.R.O.M.)

The test has proved a most useful measure of performances which involve simple but rapid coordination of eyes and hands with fine manipulative movements of the fingers. It also appears to be concerned with simple reaction time and movement time to visual stimuli, the important factors being the speed of the movement of the arm and of the fingers in grasping, placing and releasing a small object.

The apparatus consists of a large pegboard filled with four rows of cylindrical wooden blocks. It has been mainly used for two different forms of the test. The 'Placing test' is basically a measure of the rate of hand movements, and the 'Turning test' indicates the rate of finger manipulation.

Under normal circumstances the aptitude required for these actions is believed to be fully developed by the time a person has reached the age of 15 years. The standard norms are therefore applicable down to this lower age limit. This, however, does not detract from the possibilities that the test has for identifying deficiencies in the performances of children below this age. In this respect it is interesting to compare the scores of a group of children on this test and on Stott's test of motor impairment.

The mean score of a group of fifty E.S.N. children tested by Whiting *et al.* (1968), on the M.R.O.M. test, was found to be 21·1 seconds. This compares with a mean score of 28·7 obtained for thirteen (26%) of these children who failed on the manual dexterity item of Stott's test at 2 years below their own age level of 10 years. A similar discrepancy was found between the scores of a group of primary school children when the 8% who failed on the manual dexterity subtest scored significantly below the group mean on the M.R.O.M. test.

(b) Psychomotor test of speed and accuracy—Spiral Maze test (Gibson, 1964)

The effects of emotional behaviour on skilled performances has been the subject of investigations by psychologists and a talking point for educationalists and sports critics for many years. In this context the study is primarily concerned with one aspect of this vast field, namely the assessment of personality maladjustment in items of psychomotor performance.

With a view to assessing personality in psychomotor terms and for the study of behaviour disorders, Gibson (1964) has constructed a spiral maze test. It appeared as a direct descendant of the Porteus Maze test and from research into the technique that Porteus (1914) had developed for the measurement of intelligence.

Arising largely from the work of Montessori with mentally retarded children in Italy, emphasis was placed upon the need for an effective diagnostic instrument for selecting children suitable for treatment. The Binet–Simon Scale, in use at the time, was believed to have certain inadequacies in this respect as it failed to discriminate effectively between educational *potential* and previous educational experience. In response to this need Porteus developed a series of mazes of increasing difficulty and a scoring system for the evaluation of an individual's ability to carry out an appropriate sequence of steps in the achievement of an objective, namely, finding the way out of a printed labyrinth. The level of intelligence was indicated by the degree of difficulty of the mazes that the subject was able to solve.

In 1942, Porteus arrived at a standard system of scoring the *quality* of performance. A 'qualitative score' ('Q') was based upon the number and type of error (the type falling into certain categories, such as cutting the corners, touching the sides of the pathways and making slovenly wavy lines). In view of the diverse nature of the errors, whether of perceptual, cognitive or motor origins, certain doubts must exist as to the validity of a single error score. Whatever the high Q score represents, in terms of abnormalities in psycho-motor responses, there is evidence that it is a characteristic of individuals who show high neurotic tendencies (Foulds, 1951).

The link between maze test performances and neuroticism, and also with brain damage has been made by a number of workers (Benton *et al.* (1963); Elithorn *et al.* (1964); Porteus (1956)). Stott has included maze tests at certain age levels in his test of motor impairment which may be the result of minimal brain damage.

The Gibson Spiral Maze test attempts to identify characteristics in an individual's psycho-motor performance in terms of personality traits. Unlike its ancestor it is extremely quick to administer and the scoring is straightforward and reliable. The test itself measures the speed and accuracy of a motor response made under relatively stressful conditions. The 'maze' is a spiral design which presents a pathway 1·2 cm. wide and 235 cm. long, bordered by heavy black lines. A total of fifty-six 'obstacles', represented by circular dots $\frac{1}{5}$ in. in diameter, appear at random intervals along the pathway. In the strictest sense, the design is not a true maze, for there are no blind alleys or alternative paths. This excludes the memory factor involved in the 'trial and error' solution of ordinary mazes. The scoring represents both the *time* taken to draw a pencil line along the path, and the *errors* incurred by touching the obstacles or the borders. The subject is therefore required to 'trade' speed with accuracy in performing under a certain degree of stress imposed by the verbal encouragements of the examiner (given both before and during the task) to 'Go as quickly as you can!'

Using the Spiral Maze test with 100 children in primary schools, Gibson (1965) showed their performances to be related to the teachers' assessment of their general conduct in the classroom. This they classified into the categories of 'good', 'average', and 'naughty'. The distribution of both 'time' scores (indicating *quick* or *slow* performances) and the 'error' scores (showing *accurate* or *careless*) are related to these behavioural categories.

The results indicate that the 'naughty' boys clearly predominate (i.e. 40%) in the 'Quick and Careless' scoring zone, while there was a tendency for the 'good' boys to be more accurate in their responses (i.e. 32% 'Slow and Accurate', and 29% 'Quick and Accurate'). Gibson found that the *error score* was the more effective discriminator between the good and the naughty boys. He also found that this score differed significantly with other groups that included children in approved schools, and maladjusted boys in primary and secondary schools. From their performances on the spiral maze, Gibson observed a general tendency for these children to sacrifice accuracy for speed.

In a study by Whiting *et al.* (1969) it was hypothesised that this characteristic may have accounted for the relatively high incidence of motor impairment (as indicated by performances on Stott's test) that was reported by Stott (1966), and Bamber (1966). From a group of sixty-two boys aged between 11 and 14 years from a junior approved school, sixteen (27%) were regarded as being motor impaired (i.e. they either obtained a score of over 10, or a failure on any subtest at a level 2 years below their own age on Stott's test). Of this number, nine appeared in the 'slow and careless' quadrant of the Gibson Spiral Maze scatter plot and a further two were borderline cases. This relationship of motor impairment with the 'slow and careless' performances tends to reject the original hypothesis. However, it sheds some light on the possibilities of the Maze Test as an initial screening device, particularly in view of the ease and speed of its administration and scoring.

(iv) *Test of intelligence*—e.g. The Wechsler Intelligence Scale for Children—W.I.S.C. (1949)

The W.I.S.C. appeared as a development of the Wechsler–Bellevue Intelligence Scales used with adolescents and adults, with the addition of new items which extended the range of the test for children down to the age of 5 years.

The test represents a noticeable change from the traditional concept of Mental Age as being the equivalent of a mean score of a particular chronological age group. The IQ obtained from the W.I.S.C. has been standardised on scores for children in each group and any deviations in a child's IQ from retests in subsequent years gives his position relative to children *of his own age group*. This combats the common tendency of assuming that the intellectual capacity of a child with a high IQ may be the same as that of an older child of the same mental age who has a lower IQ. The W.I.S.C. also attempts to accommodate a more global view of intelligence as being part of the total personality of an individual, reflecting what Wechsler has referred to as 'traits of temperament and personality, such as persistence, drive and energy level, etc.'

The test consists of a possible twelve items which are subdivided into six Verbal and six Performance subtests. Two of these (Digit Span and Mazes) have been included as possible substitutes or additional items depending upon the time available for testing. The IQ is therefore computed on the basis of the following ten items:

Verbal	*Performance*
1. General Information	6. Picture Completion
2. General Comprehension	7. Picture Arrangement
3. Arithmetic	8. Block Design
4. Similarities	9. Object Assembly
5. Vocabulary	10. Coding or Mazes
	(from Wechsler 1949)

In addition to the full-scale IQ, therefore, both Verbal and Performance IQ's can be calculated.

The W.I.S.C. was standardised on a sample of 100 boys and 100 girls of each age group from 5–15 years. In common with the general practice the mean IQ for each age group was set at 100 with a standard deviation of 15. The different levels of intelligence have been classified in relation to educational attainment and potential intellectual development (Table 10).

TABLE 10

Intelligence classifications

IQ	Classification	Per cent included
130 and above	Very superior	2·2
120–129	Superior	6·7
110–119	Bright normal	16·1
90–109	Average	50·0
80–89	Dull normal	16·1
70–79	Borderline	6·7
69 and below	Mental defective	2·2

(from Wechsler, 1949)

The reliability correlation coefficients in Table 11 have been computed for each of the subtests in addition to the Verbal, Performance, and full-scale scores on the $7\frac{1}{2}$, $10\frac{1}{2}$ and $13\frac{1}{2}$ year samples. The relatively low correlations between the subtest scores, particularly of the younger of these groups, has prompted Wechsler (1949) to add the following note of caution when making assumptions regarding the validity of any particular subtest:

Judgements with respect to *differences* between scores on two tests of moderate reliability must be made with considerable caution—the lower the reliability of the scores, the more likelihood there is that the difference between them is due to chance rather than to any real difference in the abilities possessed by the child.

The validity of the full scale, as a measure of intelligence, has been confirmed by a number of independent investigators who have revealed high correlations between this and the

TABLE 11

Reliability correlation co-efficients (N = 200 in each age group)

	Age 7½ years r	Age 10½ years r	Age 13½ years r
Verbal score (excluding Digit Span)	0·88	0·96	0·96
Performance score (excluding Coding and Mazes)	0·86	0·89	0·90
Full-scale score (excluding Coding, Mazes and Digit Span)	0·92	0·95	0·94

(from Wechsler, 1949)

Stanford–Binet IQ, particularly in respect of the verbal scores. This important observation has been noted by Savage (1968) who, in his short review of the test, has further mentioned the fact that 'normal and superior children tend to score higher on the Stanford–Binet than on the W.I.S.C. and discrepancy in favour of the Binet is greater for brighter and younger subjects'.

One possible value of the W.I.S.C. as an initial screening device for motor impairment lies with these two representative measures of the 'full scale' intelligence. A marked discrepancy between the Verbal IQ and the Performance IQ may indicate a deficiency in either of these areas. A certain amount of variability between Verbal and Performance scores can be expected even in a normal population. In the 10½-year age group, for example, a 15 point difference would normally be recorded by as many as 20% of the population and a 20 point discrepancy in the V/P scores by 10%. From the adult intelligence scale (W.A.I.S.), Wechsler (1958) has calculated that a difference of 20 points would normally be found in only two cases out of 100 (i.e. SD of the mean difference = 10·2).

It cannot be assumed that these minority groups are all 'normal' cases. Cruickshank et al. (1961) have discussed this question of normal distribution theory in another context but their following remarks are equally pertinent at this point:

There is a logical fallacy in assuming that tests which have been standardised on a normal population and which are based on the assumption of quantitative differences can be applied to children who have specific learning disabilities, and who thus differ qualitatively from the standardised population.

It may well be that those children who have specific learning difficulties are, in fact, among the minority whose specific problems have contributed to their low scores on either the Verbal or Performance tests. Alternatively this minority may well contain the cases that Wechsler (1958) referred to as the 'false positives' who are the 'normal' subjects whose scores happen to fall within the range designated as abnormal. In connection with the W.A.I.S. he explained that 'a certain amount of this is inevitable, first because of the uncertainty of our criteria, and second because of the unreliability of our measures'.

By this reasoning it cannot be assumed that the V/P discrepancies alone are a direct indication of impairment. Due consideration must be given to the many 'extraneous' factors such as specific disabilities, deprivations, and motivational states that may be at least partly responsible for such discrepancies.

In a study of apraxic and agnostic defects in twenty-one children, Gubbay et al. (1965), using the W.I.S.C., noticed a marked discrepancy between Verbal and Performance scores, the latter being significantly lower in eighteen of the twenty-one cases. This they identified as a feature of Developmental Apraxia and Agnosia (clinical manifestations of underlying cerebral damage—apraxia referring to the executive, and agnosia to the cognitive disorders). Although those 'praxis' and 'gnosis' disorders result in clumsiness of physical performance (Orton, 1937), they are closely associated with involuntary movement. They are seen to be clearly distinct from the more obvious effects of deep cortical lesions (of pyramidal and extrapyramidal nerve cells) or cerebellar dysfunction, which give rise to uncoordinated voluntary motor activity. These observations were entirely supported by the findings of Walton et al. (1962) who believed that it was impossible to distinguish completely between apraxia and agnosia because the 'gnosic' defects of recognition almost invariably lead to defects of 'praxis', or execution.

Apart from the intelligence of these children other possible facets of motor impairment were observed either in dressing or constructional apraxia, the most common manifestation of the latter being poor handwriting. It is often only as a result of intelligence tests, and perhaps the observant eye of a teacher, that children with impaired neural function are identified. The work of the local Child Guidance Centres is very largely concerned with these cases.

In a study by Whiting *et al.* (1969), reported earlier in connection with the validation of Stott's test of motor impairment, the ten children who were attending a Child Guidance Centre for remedial teaching were selected for investigation because references to their 'clumsiness' had been made by either their parents, teachers or examining psychologists. It appeared to be significant that each of these children had recorded a performance score of more than 10 points lower than their verbal score on the W.I.S.C. Out of these ten cases, four were identified by Stott's test as showing a marked degree of motor impairment (i.e. they failed at least one item at a point 2 years below their own age level and/or they achieved a score of 10 or more).

These four children were then examined by a paediatrician on the following points:

(*a*) Muscle tone and power   (*e*) Position sense
(*b*) Muscle strength   (*f*) Vibration sense
(*c*) Tendon reflexes   (*g*) Pain sense.
(*d*) Coordination

From his examination no significant abnormalities were revealed, other than one case of 'slight coordination tremor', one of 'slight Pes Cavus', and another case in which the child's coordination was reported to be 'moderate'. In this particular instance, therefore, the discrepancy between Verbal and Performance scores, although relatively small, did not appear to be related to their record of motor impairment on Stott's test.

(v) *Test of perceptual abilities*
The Developmental test of Visual Perception (Frostig, 1963) arose out of investigations and observations of children who had been referred to the Marianne Frostig School of Educational Therapy because of learning difficulties. From their performances on the Bender-Gestalt, Goodenough, and other similar tests it was

believed that many of these difficulties could be attributed to disturbances in visual and auditory perception. More specific difficulties, mainly concerned with reading and writing skills, were then observed to be related to weaknesses in certain relatively independent aspects of visual perception.

From these observations, Frostig (1961) selected for her test the following five aspects of visual perception on the firm belief that, 'there should be specific relationships between them and a child's ability to learn and adjust', and that they, 'seemed to have particular relevance to school performance'.

(i)   Eye-motor coordination.
(ii) Figure-ground perception.
(iii) Form constancy.
(iv) Position in space.
(v)   Spatial relations.

A child's scores on each of these five subtests are recorded on a 'basic score sheet'. Those falling below the mean for his age group are positioned in a column which designates both the area and the extent to which 'training is needed'. His scores are therefore measured against those of the 2,100 children aged between 3 and 9 years that provided the normative data in the 1963 standardisation. This information has been used to formulate an educational programme appropriate to the individual strengths and weaknesses of each child.

(i) The tests of eye-hand coordination are concerned with the ability to coordinate vision with movements of the hand. The individual items involve drawing straight and curved lines between boundaries of decreasing width, and a straight line joining two given points.

Disabilities in this area are seen to be more directly related to difficulties in learning and performing simple visual-motor skills. They may also contribute to the poor self-concept in many of the children who lack the ability of their peers in games and other activities of high prestige value.

(ii) The assessment of figure-ground perception incorporates the ability to selectively attend to the relevant cues (i.e. the figure) in a display of confusing patterns, while disregarding all the irrelevant stimuli as background.

Frostig (1964) has suggested that a child with poor figure-ground differentiation is inclined to be inattentive and easily distracted. He may also be identified as having difficulty in initiating a new response because of his tendency to cling to the original stimulus and to repeat his previous performance. His behaviour on the test has been explained by Frostig who stated that, 'he is unable to draw a straight line between boundaries because one of the boundaries captures his attention and he directs his pencil towards and along it'.

(iii) The perception of form constancy is associated with the 'ability to perceive an object as possessing invariant properties, such as shape, position, and size in spite of the variability of the impressions on the sensory surface'.

The test involves the discrimination of a set of simple geometric shapes that are presented in different sizes and positions and in different settings.

Frostig has indicated that disabilities in this aspect, particularly in recognising the 'shape' and 'size' characteristics of an object, may present a major learning problem. A letter or a number may be difficult to recognise when displayed in a slightly unfamiliar manner. A child with these disabilities may be reluctant to catch a tennis-ball because he is unable to recognise it as such at a distance. He may wrongly identify an object because it possesses a particular quality that he has associated with something else. Therefore, a bus may be mistaken for a fire-engine simply because of its colour.

(iv) The perception of the position of an object in space (directionality) is dependent on a highly developed sense of body awareness. The observer becomes the point of reference from which the object is located on the various coordinates of 'left' or 'right', 'above' or 'below', etc.

A child lacking in body awareness may have difficulty in understanding these positional and directional terms. Frostig has pointed out that his reading and handwriting may contain many reversals and inversions. 'He will read "was" for "saw", and "on" for "no", "w" for "m" and 24 for 42 because the right and the left and the up and down of these will have no significance for him.'

For the assessment of this ability a child is required to differentiate between sets of drawings of common objects (e.g. a chair) by identifying a reversal or rotation.

(v) The perception of spatial relations includes the ability to see the positional relationships between objects. This appears to be a development of the ability of the observer to locate the objects in relation to himself (i.e. 'position in space'). Frostig has explained 'You must be able to recognise that an object is in front of you before you are able to understand that one object is in front of another.'

The tests that she has chosen to assess this ability involve copying a set of patterns (of increasing complexity) consisting of horizontal, vertical and oblique lines that connect a series of dots.

Disabilities in this area may be observed as mistakes in a child's reading and handwriting where he has failed to reproduce the correct sequence of letters in a word, or words in a sentence. Frostig has taken this a stage further by stating that a child with a spatial relations problem 'will have difficulty in following a story or television programme and will be unable to reproduce it in its proper sequence'.

From the original test, produced in 1959, certain modifications were made with the intention of providing a series of items of increasing difficulty in each of the five subtests. This progression was in accordance with the evidence of the development of these areas of visual perception in children from the age of 3 to approximately $7\frac{1}{2}$ years. It enabled the calculation of the perceptual age and perceptual quotient of the child to be introduced in the overall assessment.

The perceptual age indicates the developmental level on each and all of these abilities regardless of the chronological age of the child. From the data provided by the 1963 standardisation a raw score of 8, for example, on subtest 1 was established as 'normal' for a child aged 4 years 9 months, and the score of a 'normal' child aged 7 years 3 months on the same test, was found to be 16. Tables are also provided for the conversion of raw scores to scale scores and scale scores to perceptual quotients for the various chronological age groups from 4 to 8 years. The scale scores have been computed by dividing the perceptual age by the chronological age, and multiplying by 10. The quotient represents the sum of the scale scores for each of the five subtests. The median for this has been set at 100, with quotients of 110 and 90 representing the 75th and 25th percentile ranks respectively. Children whose perceptual quotients appear in the lower quartile (i.e. below 90) have been regarded as in need of special training.

N

Frostig has explained that all of these three measures (perceptual quotients, subtest perceptual scores, and scale scores) must be taken into account in any assessment of a child's level of perceptual ability. For children over the age of 10, however, the subtest perceptual age equivalent has been regarded as a more accurate predictive index than the perceptual quotient or the scale scores. It has also been recognised that the test performances of the older children may be contaminated by the influence of other maturational abilities and the acquisition of related perceptual-motor skills.

In a test–re-test study of reliability involving fifty children with learning difficulties, Frostig *et al.* (1961) found a correlation of 0·98 between the perceptual quotients after an interval of 3 weeks. In a later study, conducted under slightly different testing conditions in which 144 first and second grade children were retested after an interval of two weeks, the correlation was found to be 0·8. A wide discrepancy was seen to exist between the test–re-test correlations on each of the subtests taken by the first grade children (the range extended from a correlation of 0·33 for the Eye-motor coordination tests, to 0·83 for the tests of Form Constancy). No evidence has been put forward to account for this discrepancy.

An assessment of the validity of the test was also reported by Frostig (1964). This study took the form of a comparison of the scores of 374 kindergarten children with the teachers' ratings of 'classroom adjustment', 'motor coordination' and 'intellectual functioning'. On each of these aspects of the children's behaviour the chi-square comparisons with their scores on the test proved to be significant at the 0·001 level. This offers a small but encouraging piece of evidence to support Frostig's thesis that disturbances in a child's visual perception, as measured by the test, are likely to have an adverse effect upon his educational progress. In support of the test both for its screening and diagnostic values, Frostig *et al.* (1964) have stated:

> Testing of these abilities not only permits the measuring of specific assets and liabilities but also allows the exploration of the relationships between these abilities and school achievement. Moreover, the relationship of these abilities to each other and to various personality measures may prove to be of diagnostic significance.

References

Abercrombie, M. L. J., Gardiner, P. A., Hansen, E., Jonckheere, J., Lindon, R. L., Solomon, G. & Tyson, M. C. (1964) Visual, perceptual and visuo-motor impairment in physically handicapped children. *Percept. & Motor Skills*, 18, 561–625.

Anthony, H. S. (1960) Anxiety as a function of psycho-motor and social behaviour. *Brit. J. Psych.*, 51, 141–152.

Bamber, J. (1966) Unpublished thesis. Psychology Department, University of Glasgow.

Bender, A. L. (1938) A visual-motor Gestalt test. *Res. Monog.* New York; Amer. Orthopsychiatric Assn.

Benton, A., Elithorn, A., Fagel, M. L. & Kerr, M. (1963) A perceptual maze test sensitive to brain damage. *J. Neurol. Neurosurg. Psychiat.*, 26, 540–544.

Carey, R. A. Comparison of the Lincoln Revision of the Oseretzky test of motor proficiency with selected motor ability tests. University of Indiana. Unpublished thesis.

Cassell, R. (1949) Vineland adaption of the Oseretzky tests. *Training School Bulletin*, supp. to vol. 43, 3–4.

Clarke, T. A., Johnson, G. B., Morris, P. R. & Page, M. (1968) *Motor Impairment. A study of clumsy children.* Unpublished dissertation. University of Leeds Institute of Education.

Cowan, E. A. & Pratt, B. M. (1934) The hurdle jump as a developmental and diagnostic test of motor coordination for children. *Child. Dev.*, 5, 107–121.

Cruickshank, W. M., Bentzen, F. A., Ratzeburg, F. H. & Tannhauser, M. T. (1961) *A Teaching Method for Brain injured and Hyperactive Children.* Syracuse University Press.

Decroly, J. & Bratu, E. A. (1934) The measurement of motor functions in children and adolescents, *Rev. Pedog.*, 4, 12.

Doll, E. A. (1946) The Oseretzky Scale. *Amer. J. of Ment. Def.*, 50, 485–487.

Doll, E. A. (1946) The Oseretzky tests. *Training School Bulletin*, 43, 1.

Doll, E. A. (1946) *The Oseretzky Tests of Motor Performance.* Minneapolis Educational Trust Bureau.

Doll, E. A. & Walker, M. S. (1941) Handedness in cerebral palsied children. *J. Consult. Psych.*, 5, 9–17.

Elithorn, A., Jones, D., Kerr, M. & Lee, D. (1964) The effects of the variation of two physical parameters on empirical difficulty in a perceptual task. *Brit. J. Psych.*, 55, 31–37.

Espenschade, A. (1940) Motor performance in adolescence. *Monog. Soc. Res. Child Devel.*, 5, 1.

Fairweather, D. V. & Illsley, R. (1960) Obstetric and social origins of mentally handicapped children. *Brit. J. of Prev. Soc. Med.*, 14, 149–159.

Field, J. (1960) Two types of tables for use with Wechsler's intelligence. *J. Clin. Psych.*, 16, 3–7.

Fish, B. (1961) The study of motor development in infancy and its relation to psychological functioning. *Amer. J. of Psychiat.*, 17, 1113–1118.

Fisher, M. (1956) Left hemiplegia and motor impersistence. *J. Nerv. Ment. Dis.*, 123, 201–218.

Foster, F. C. (1930) Significant response in certain memory tests. *J. App. Psych.*, 4, 142–154.

Foulds, G. A. (1951) Temperamental differences in maze performance. *Brit. J. Psych.*, 4, 142–154.

Frostig, M., Lefever, D. W. & Whittlesey, J. R. B. (1961) A developmental test of visual perception for evaluating normal and neurologically handicapped children. *Percept. Motor Skills*, 12, 383–389.

Frostig, M. (1963) *Developmental Test of Visual Perception.* California: Consulting Psychologists' Press.

Frostig, M. & Horne, D. (1964) *The Frostig program for the development of visual perception.* Chicago: Follet.

Frostig, M., Lefever, D. W. & Whittlesey, J. R. B. (1964) *Developmental Test of Visual Perception* (3rd Edition). Palo Alto, California: Consulting Psychologists' Press.

Frostig, M., Maslow, P., Lefever, D. W. & Whittlesey, J. R. B. (1964) *The Marianne Frostig Developmental Test of Visual Perception. 1963. Standardisation.* Palo Alto, California: Consulting Psychologists' Press.

Garfield, J. C. (1964) Motor impersistence in normal and brain damaged children. *Neurology*, 14, 623–630.

Garfield, J. C., Benton, A. L. & McQueen, J. C. (1966) Motor impersistence in brain damaged and cultural-familial defectives. *J. Nerv. Ment. Dis.*, 142, 434–440.

Garrett, E. S., Price, A. C. & Deabler, H. L. (1957) Diagnostic testing for cortical brain impairment. A.M.A. *Arch. Neurol. Psychiat.*, 77, 223–225.

Gesell, A. (1941) *The first five years of life.* London: Methuen.

Gesell, A. & Amatruda, C. S. (1941). *Development Diagnosis.* New York: Hoeber.

Gibson, H. B. (1964) The Spiral Maze, a psychomotor test with implications for the study of delinquency. *Brit. J. of Psych.*, 54, 219–225.

Gibson, H. B. (1965) *Manual of the Gibson Spiral Maze.* London: University Press.

Graham, F. K. & Kendall, S. (1960) Memory for Designs. *Percept. & Motor Skills*, 11, 147–188.

Graham, F. K. & Kendall, B. S. (1946) Performance of brain damaged cases on a Memory for Design test. *J. of Abnormal Soc. Psych.*, 41, 303–314.

Graham, F. K. & Kendall, S. (1947) A note on the scoring of the Memory for Design test. *J. of Abnormal Soc. Psych.*, 42, 253.

Goodenough, F. L. (1926) *Measurement of intelligence by drawings.* New York: Harcourt, Brace & World.

Gubbay, S. S., Ellis, E., Walton, J. J. & Court, S. D. M. (1965) A study of apraxic and agnostic defects in 21 children. *Brain*, 88, 295.

Harris, B. (1963) *Children's Drawings as Measures of Intellectual Maturity.* New York: Harcourt, Brace & World.

Heath, R. S. (1944) Clinical significance of motor defectives with military implications. *Amer. J. of Psych.*, 57, 481–499.

Heath, R. S. (1953) Relation of railwalking and other motor performance of mental defectives to mental age and aetiological type. *Training School Bulletin*, 50, 119–127.

Hildreth, G. & Griffiths, N. L. (1946) *Metropolitan Readiness Test.* Yonkers-on-Hudson: World Book Co.

Juarros, C. (1939) Practical value of Oseretzky's group tests for determining motor age. *Psicetecnia*, 1, 40–60.

Joynt, R. J., Benton, A. L. & Fogel, M. L. (1962) Behavioural and pathological correlations of motor impersistence. *Neurology*, 12, 876–881.

Kinsbourne, M. & Warrington, E. K. (1963) Developmental factors in reading and writing backwardness. *Brit. J. of Psych.*, 54, 145–156.

Knobloch, H. & Pasamanik, B. (1960) The developmental behavioural approach to the neurologic examination in infancy. *Child Dev.*, 33, 181–198.

Kolburne, L. L. (1965) Effective Education for the Mentally Retarded Children. New York: Vintage.

Kopp, H. (1943) The relationship of stuttering to motor disturbance. *Nerv. Child*, 2, 107–116.

Koppitz, E. M. (1958) The Bender Gestalt test and learning disturbances in young children. *J. Clin. Psych.*, 14, 292–295.

Lassner, R. (1948) Annotated bibliography of the Oseretzky test of motor performance. *J. of Consult. Psych.*, 12, 37–47.

Machover, K. (1949) *Personality projection in the drawing of the human figure.* Springfield: Thomas.

McCloy, C. H. (1934) The measurement of general motor capacity and general motor ability. *Res. Quart.*, 5, 46–61.

Meredith, P. (1964) Decisions—theory in the light of recent research. Unpublished paper, Dept. of Psychology, University of Leeds.

Metheny, E. (1938) Studies of the Johnson test as a test of motor educability. *Res. Quart.*, 9, 105–114.

Miller, L. C., Lowenfeld, R., Linder, R. & Turner, J. (1963) Reliability of Koppitz' scoring system for the Bender Gestalt. *J. Clin. Psych.*, 19, 2111.

Muscio, B. (1922)   Motor capacity with special reference to vocational guidance. *Brit. J. of Psych.*, 13, 157–184.

Oseretzky, N. A. (1923)   Metric scale for studying the motor capacity of children, published in Russian. Referred to in Rudolph Lassner Annotated Bibliography of the Oseretzky Test of Motor Proficiency. *J. of Consult. Psych.*, 1948, 12, 37–47.

Oseretzky, N. A. and Guerewitch, M. O. (1965)   Concerning methods of examining the motor functions. *Mschr. Psychiat. Neurol.*, 59, 37–103.

Oseretzky, N. A. (1929)   A group method of examining the motor functions of children and adolescents. *Z. Kinderforsch*, 35, 352–372.

Oseretzky, N. A. & Guerewitch, M. O. (1930)   Constitutional variations in psychomotor ability. *Arch. Psychiat. Nervenkr.*, 9, 286–312.

Pascall, C. R. & Suttell, B. S. (1951)   *The Bender Gestalt Test.* New York: Grune & Stratton.

Perrin, F. A. C. (1921)   An experimental study of motor ability. *J. Exp. Psych.*, 4, 24–56.

Porteus, S. D. (1942)   *Qualitative performance in the Maze Test.* Vineland: Smith.

Porteus, S. D. (1956)   *Porteus Maze Test of Intelligence.* California: Pacific Books.

Porteus, S. D. (1959)   *The Maze Test and Clinical Psychology.* California: Pacific Books.

Prechtl, H. F. R. & Stemmer, C. J. (1962)   The Choreiform syndrome in children. *Dev. Med. & Child Neurol.*, 4, 119–127.

Rutter, M., Graham, P. & Birch, D. (1966)   Intercorrelations between the choreiform syndrome, reading disability and psychiatric disorders. *Dev. Med. & Child Neurol.*, 8, 149–159.

Savage, D. R. (1968)   *Psychometric Assessment of the Individual Child.* Harmondsworth: Penguin.

Seashore, R. H. (1928)   Selecting individuals best suited for training or work in practical motor skills. *Psych. Monog.*, 30, 51–66.

Seashore, R. H. (1930)   Individual differences in motor skills. *J. Genet. Psych.*, 3, 33–66.

Sloan, W. (1955)   The Lincoln/Oseretzky motor development scale. *Gen. Psych. Monog.*, 51, 183–252.

Spreen, O. & Benton, A. L. (1965)   Comparative studies of some psychological tests of cerebral damage. *J. Nerv. Ment. Disease*, 5, 323–333.

Stott, D. H. (1964)   Why maladjustment. *New Society*, Dec. 10th.

Stott, D. H. (1966)   A general test of motor impairment for children. *Dev. Med. and Child Neurol.*, 8, 523–531.

Stott, D. H., Moyes, F. A. & Headridge, S. E. (1966)   Test of motor impairment. Dept. of Psychol., University of Glasgow.

Stott, D. H. (1966)   *Studies of Troublesome Children.* London: Tavistock.

Stott, D. H. (1966)   A general test of motor impairment for children. *Dev. Med. Child Neurol.*, 8, 523–531.

Stott, D. H. (1966) Three years to study the 'Ham Fisted'. *The Times Educ. Suppl.*, April.

Strauss, A. A. & Lehtinen, L. C. (1948) *Psycopathology and education of the brain injured child.* New York: Grune & Stratton.

Thams, R. (1955) A factor analysis of the Lincoln/Oseretzky motor development scale. Unpublished dissertation, University of Michigan.

Thweatt, R. C. (1963) Prediction of school learning disabilities through the use of the Bender Gestalt test. *J. Clin. Psych.*, 19, 216–217.

Vandenburg, S. G. (1964) Factor analytic study of the Lincoln/Oseretzky test of motor proficiency. *Percept. & Motor Skills*, 19, 23–41.

Van der Lugt, M. J. A. (1939) *Un profil psychomoteur.* Paris Auber (Editions Montaigne).

Walton, J. J., Ellis, E. & Court, S. D. N. (1962) Clumsy children. Developmental apraxia and agnosia. *Brain*, 85, 603.

Wechsler, D. (1949) *Wechsler Intelligence Scale for Children. Manual.* New York: The Psychological Corporation.

Wechsler, D. (1958) *The measurement and appraisal of adult intelligence.* London, Baltiere, Tindall.

Whiting, H. T. A., Clarke, T. A. & Morris, P. R. (1969) A clinical validation of the Stott test of motor impairment. *Br. J. of Soc. Clin. Psych.*, 8, 270–274.

Whiting, H. T. A., Davies, J. G., Gibson, J. M., Lumley, R., Sutcliffe, R. S. E. & Morris, P. R. (1969) *Motor Impairment in an Approved School Population.* Unpublished paper, Physical Education Dept., Leeds University.

Witkin, H. A. (1959) The perception of the upright. Reprinted from *Scientific American.* San Francisco: Freeman.

Witkin, H. A., Dyk, R. B., Faterson, H. F., Goodenough, D. R. & Karp, S. A. (1962) *Psychological differentiation.* New York: Wiley.

Wood, I. & Shulman, E. (1940) The Ellis visual design test. *J. Ed. Psych.*, 31, 591–602.

Yarmolenko, A. (1933) The motor sphere of school age children. *J. Genet. Psych.*, 42, 398–316.

Yule, W. (1967) A short form of the Oseretzky test of motor proficiency. Paper read at Annual Conference of Brit. Psychol Society, Belfast. April.

Yule, W., Graham, P. & Tizard, J. (1967) Motor impersistence in 9 year old children. Unpublished paper, Dept. of Child Devel., Univ. of London.

CHAPTER 7

Compensatory Education

> *The treatment of learning difficulties is admittedly a complex task. The symptoms are commonly multiple, their causes are commonly multiple, and the treatment procedures, to be fully effective, must usually be multiple. But as we begin to understand better the meaning of our evaluations, and to devise and experiment with more techniques, we hope we will gain a deeper understanding of the underlying difficulties of children and know better how to provide for each child the programme that will enable him to achieve his maximum potential.*
>
> (Frostig, 1969)

Behavioural characteristics associated with disturbances in perceptual-motor functions

Distractibility

Every activity (writing, reading and kicking a ball, etc.) is performed against a background of extraneous visual, auditory, and tactile impressions. The performance of a normal child in this natural situation has been summed up by Pedder (1964):

> In the normal individual the stimulus situation and response possibilities are coordinated and patterned in such a manner that organised rational behaviour or meaningful activity results.

Normal perceptual and conceptual activity is concerned with discriminating and largely ignoring those aspects of the whole stimulus situation which are not relevant to the task in hand, in order that the responses of the individual will not be affected by them. In responding to extraneous visual or auditory stimuli the individual's attention is distracted. According to Vernon (1962):

> Fluctuations of attention depend to a greater or lesser extent upon conditions within the individual himself—general health, state of fatigue, interest in his task and strength of motivation for maintaining attention.

The difficulties that a child may have in selecting and organising the relevant information and in disregarding that which is unimportant suggests that he may be easily distracted. The attention of the child may be attracted by an irrelevant background detail which would normally be disregarded. This lack of concern for the essentials often gives the impression of inattentiveness, whereas the child may be hypersensitive and extremely attentive to detail. The child may be unable to concentrate his attention for any length of time on a particular object in his environment. He is constantly being diverted by everything around him, by the activity of others and by normally inconspicuous background stimuli. An example of this type of behaviour was referred to by Gesell & Amatruda (1941):

> Such a child not only attends to the noise outside but is unable to inhibit the impulse to go to the window to find it.

Strauss & Kephart (1955) referred to the effect of any extraneous stimulus as bringing about a 'condition of momentary disequilibrium' until it has been satisfactorily identified. When this has been done attention returns to the situation at hand. Cratty (1969) associated this behaviour with:

> The persistence of an immature stage of development during which time the child feels compelled to inspect everything around him.

He has also proposed the theory of a breakdown in any one of the several stages in the perceptual-motor process to account for the hyperactive behaviour which is a characteristic of these distractible children. In more specific terms he has tentatively placed the disturbance at the perceptual level, by reference to the 'selection-rejection system' in which he suggests that the child 'may be attempting to handle too many stimuli'. A somewhat different view of this behaviour has been proposed by Signy (1960) who observed that many children in E.S.N.

schools were unable to persist with a task the moment that a problem arose. He suggested that this could not always be explained by a short attention span and was more likely the result of a sheltering and over-indulgent parental attitude that encouraged the children to avoid those activities which they found difficult to perform.

Floyer (1955), referring to the behaviour of a group of cerebral palsied children, found that the distractibility in some cases, even among children who were not educationally retarded, was so marked that they were unable to hold their attention on any task long enough to achieve even minor success. Cruickshank & Dolphin (1951) believed that distractibility and the associated short attention span accounted for the poor reproduction of the drawings, block patterns, and marble board designs that formed the basis of the tests that he used with brain-injured children. They also observed that some of the children showed an inability to concentrate their attention upon any one object. Their reaction was equally strong to all factors in the immediate environment. They referred to this characteristic as 'forced responsiveness'. It was thought to be related to the figure-ground differentiation problem in which the background and foreground stimuli were received with similar intensity.

Disinhibition

The problems of forced responsiveness and distractibility are closely associated with what has been defined by Strauss & Kephart (1955), Cruickshank et al. (1961), and others, as the characteristic of 'disinhibition'. The behaviour of a normal child in any situation is often the result of a choice that he has made between several possible responses. At a conceptual level he is often able to consider and evaluate the consequences of his actions and to select the response which he judges to be the most suitable. As a result of these decisions at a non-overt level, the child has rejected or 'inhibited' certain responses in a choice situation.

The distractible child may have difficulty in perceiving the relationships between the various impressions of a given situation. His assessment of a situation may therefore be inaccurate. He may have difficulty in evaluating the consequences of his actions.

This behaviour is reflected in what Cruickshank *et al.* (1961) have described as,

> the failure of the child to refrain from response to any stimuli which produces motor activity, e.g. holes into which fingers can be poked, cracks in a desk which can be traced with a pencil or a finger.

Strauss & Kephart (1955) have discussed the possible causes of these difficulties in the following way:

> Both perceptually and conceptually he is operating on less material at any one time than is the normal individual. . . . Instead of a choice among many responses, he has available only one response.

At times the child appears to be unable to avoid what is almost a spontaneous or impulsive reaction to certain stimuli. Such behaviour is characterised by a greater intensity of response. In his reaction to certain stimuli and in the accomplishment of a given task, he appears to expend far more energy than a normal child.

In a group situation, behaviour of this nature creates a problem when, as is often the case, the disinhibited responses are socially disapproved. In addition, they are the unexpected reactions which usually attract the most attention.

Perseveration

The difficulty that certain children have in shifting their attention from one activity or concept to another has been noted by Goldstein (1936), Werner (1941), Strauss & Lehtinen (1948), Caldwell (1956), Tansley & Gulliford (1962) and others. It has been described as a symptom of neural dysfunction that is closely associated with forced responsiveness, and referred to as 'perseveration'.

A child may be so absorbed in a particular activity that he appears to be oblivious to all other aspects of his environment. Goldstein observed that this occurred when the child who had achieved a successful response tended not only to cling to the original stimulus but also to repeat his performance many times. Cruickshank *et al.* (1961) interpreted this in terms of 'the apparent inertia of the organism' in its response, this being the result of a prolonged 'after-effect' of the particular stimulus to which the child has made an adjustment.

MOTOR IMPAIRMENT AND COMPENSATORY EDUCATION

This would perhaps explain the apparent paradox between
a child's undue fixation occurring after a satisfactory performance and, at the same time, his abnormal distractibility.

When confronted with a new task, particularly one which he
finds difficult, a child may continue to repeat the original
performance. Strauss & Werner (1942) found a similar response
in the performance of several brain injured children in tests
of Memory for Design. When asked to recall the more complicated designs, that were in the form of dot patterns on a series
of cards, they continually reproduced the last design that they
had successfully remembered. On the more difficult design they
made 20% perseverations in all trials. On the same test a paired
control group of eighteen non-brain-damaged children made
no perseverations.

Goldstein (1962) cites the following example of this in a more
conventional learning situation:

> A child who is writing seems unable to initiate a new sequence
> of acts and repeats the letter he has just completed.

In reading, the visual impressions and associations of a
particular word may be so demanding of a child's attention that
they influence his recognition of the succeeding word. In
Physical Education a child may repeat a well-practised movement even after he has been asked to finish the activity.

Counteractive measures

Tansley & Gulliford (1962) believe that this tendency to repeat
familiar activities helps to provide an increased sense of security,
and partly accounts for the good rote memory which brain
injured children often show in their ability to recall numerical
tables and poems, etc. The fact that many children with these
learning problems have extreme difficulty in concentrating
their attention for any length of time suggests that they may
progress more satisfactorily with relatively short and varied
periods of work. In more specific terms, Gesell & Amatruda
(1941) have suggested ways in which the efforts of the educator
can be directed to help minimise the effects of this distractible
and hyperactive form of behaviour. These included the manipulation and control of the external environment of the learning
situation. In restricting the over-stimulating conditions of a
normal classroom by structuring the environment to exclude the

distraction of pictures, unnecessary noises, and movement, etc., a child may be encouraged to concentrate more of his attention on the task in hand. Where more space is required for physical education lessons, Cratty (1969) reports having greater success with some hyperactive and distractible children when working in indoor handball courts, where the conditions have a less disturbing effect upon skill performance.

In discussing the effects of this type of structured environment, Gesell & Amatruda (1941) observed:

> With decreased interference from the general disturbances comes an increased responsiveness to the learning situation. Control of behaviour makes learning possible; knowledge gained makes possible more effective control of behaviour. . . . As the disturbances are lessened, the protections are gradually removed, for direction of a child's behaviour should eventually be effected from within himself rather than from externally regulated conditions.

In an attempt to *prolong* a child's attention, Cratty has experimented with the use of certain absorbing activities such as balancing on a wooden rocker. These have a natural appeal to the child and can be made progressively more challenging by the imposition of competitive standards. Other measures include techniques that Cratty has adopted from the work of Jacobson (1938) in an attempt to help the hyperactive child to consciously relax. These exercises, performed either sitting at a desk or lying down, involve tensing and relaxing various parts of the body. The purpose of these is to instill in the child an awareness of the effects of excess energies and muscular tensions.

Other conditions that have been experimented with in regard to these problems have been outlined by Francis-Williams (1964). From the results of her work with distractible children she emphasised the value of the following:

(i) The importance of a well-defined and limited framework within which the child is expected to work.
(ii) The use of teaching materials that intensify the stimulus in terms of figure and ground.
(iii) The use of materials that help the child to relate isolated parts to form a patterned whole.

While supporting the prevalent idea of providing working conditions in which the environmental stimuli are strongly reduced, she mentions that this idea of 'protection' is somewhat controversial. This view is also supported by Schaffer (1958). In his observations of babies under 7 months of age who had been in hospital for periods of up to 2 weeks, he noticed that for some time after their discharge they appeared to be almost unaware of objects and people, including their own mothers. They were described as having become 'rigidified and set in the unchanging perceptual environment of the hospital ward'. It was suggested from this evidence that normal concentration, perception, and thought could only be maintained in a constantly changing environment. Francis-Williams describes this as a possible example of 'sensory deprivation', in which the 'capacity to concentrate deteriorates and attention fluctuates and lapses'. This is mentioned as an important consideration in the educational provision made for the child showing signs of distractible behaviour.

A measure of the possible success of an approach which also aimed to reduce extraneous stimuli may be judged from the work of Cruickshank et al. (1961). They selected a group of forty children, whose average age was 8 years, with a mean IQ of 80, on the basis of their reported learning difficulties. The children were also found to have behaviour characteristics of distractibility, disinhibition, dissociation, disturbance in figure-ground relationship, perseveration, and poor body image. These were considered to be of organic origin, although neither the existence nor the degree of neurological impairment in some cases had been positively established. A noticeable feature of the behaviour of these children was their proneness to minor accidents. Cruickshank recorded;

> Even the most ordinary movements are unpredictable and liable to cause mishaps. Frequently someone stumbles even in walking across a room.

In spite of their apparently 'normal' physical appearance, both their movement vocabulary and choice of activities was described as being below the level of other children of the same age. Their preference for certain toys, for example, was more characteristic of children in first grade or even in nursery school.

Cruickshank was concerned with the child's functioning in a learning situation and the means of improving his rate of progress. In this respect, he considered the findings of neurological examinations to be only of limited value to any solution of these learning problems. The forty children were divided into four matched groups of ten. Two of these were made the control groups and received conventional teaching methods for one year. Over the same period the other two groups were taught by an experimental teaching method which involved the following:

(i) Reduced environmental stimuli and space.

To avoid the distractions of a normal classroom situation, Cruickshank suggested that the smallest practical area is that required for the child's chair and desk. This not only provided for individual teaching but also created what was believed to be a more secure environment for the child to work in.

(ii) A structured teaching programme and school routine.

This involved the simplifying and restructuring of the learning environment in order to provide the hyperactive child with more opportunity for experiencing the successes that had escaped him in the past. Cruickshank identified success with the 'positive conditioning' that underlies the learning process.

(iii) Increased stimulus value of the teaching materials (e.g. bright and distinctive colouring in order to facilitate the focus of attention).

The main feature of Cruickshank's approach to the education of these hyperactive children was his restructuring of the educational situation. This was based upon their special needs, as determined by the past school and medical records, and their learning difficulties which were manifest in these behavioural characteristics of distractibility, and perseveration, etc. By this means, therefore, he aimed to take into account the psychopathology of the child and to direct attention to the disability by using the child's strengths to correct his weaknesses. Cruickshank advocated the principle of leading the child, 'through the things he cannot do—step by step up the developmental ladder'.

This work of compensatory education was aimed to begin at the level where the child was able to succeed. The rate of progress was determined by his successive achievements. Thus, the child was carefully guided in his experience of those activities which he may have missed at an earlier age. Cruickshank has repeatedly emphasised this need to 'fill in the gaps' of a child's vocabulary of experiences which are a necessary part of the normal maturational process. Referring to these experiences as 'the usual developmental activities', he pointed out:

> The fact that they did not do them and the knowledge of the ones they skipped are matters of great importance in bringing such children up-to-date in academic areas.

The result of his teaching methods after one year with the group of forty children were reported to be encouraging. The 'experimental' classes had made temporary gains in comparison with the control group, particularly in their scores on tests of visual perception. The difference in the recorded progress of the two groups, however, was observed to be small and these earlier gains were nullified at the end of the second year after the groups had been mixed.

Learning difficulties associated with disturbances in perceptual-motor functions

The performances of slow-learning children on psychological tests that have been used by Werner (1944), Wechsler (1949), Benton (1950), Cruickshank (1951), Bender (1952), Frostig (1963), Kephart (1965) and others, have revealed certain disabilities which are believed to handicap the learning process. These are represented by deviations in the standard of performance which is generally below that of a normal child.

A motor impaired child may show disturbances in perception, concept formation, and in executive or effector responses, either separately or in combination.

In terms of the Gestalt psychology, perception can be described as having two aspects. The first is the psychological process in which part of a 'whole' is seen or heard or felt in relationship to the other parts. The whole consists of the integration of all of the parts into a unique entity, which represents more than their mere summation. In normal perceptual activity the 'whole' or object is immediately recognised and acquires meaning and significance. The sight of a common object such as a chair is recognised at a glance without any detailed examination of its composite parts.

Some children are often more attracted to the details of an object and may have difficulty in perceiving their relationship with each other and with the whole. In this case, the whole is seen more as a collection of parts rather than something unique with qualities of its own. This characteristic was observed by Strauss & Kephart (1955) in the test performances of a number of brain injured children:

> They are able to perceive the parts but do not combine them adequately into wholes. Thus in drawing a square they are apt to leave the corners unconnected. The lines are independent of one another and independent of the whole.

The second area of perception concerns the recognition of a 'whole' as a foreground figure against a background. In normal perception, only those impressions which are regarded as being important or meaningful are selected from the wide field of sensory stimuli. These become the foreground figure and all other impressions are ignored as irrelevant background material.

Psychological tests have been devised to reflect disturbances in the perceptual activity that may relate to some of the difficulties that certain children encounter in the learning process (particularly in relation to the acquisition of visual-motor skills). Commonly used tests have been those which require a child to identify or reproduce various geometric designs. Simple shapes are presented against a structured background, or embedded with other shapes into a patterned figure.

Some children may have difficulty in recalling the original shapes either by copying, matching, or visualising them. The difficulties are seen to increase as the patterning of the background becomes more involved.

This observation was recorded by Miller & Rosenfeld (1952) in a study of cerebral palsied children. They stated that the lack of ability to recall such forms was evident even though some of the children appeared to have the necessary coordination and mental ability to do so.

In everyday learning situations, it is necessary not only to obtain clear recognition of an object, but also to perceive its significance and relationship to other relevant foreground objects in the sensory field. In this connection Strauss & Lehtinen (1948) found that some brain damaged children are more likely than normal children to associate objects because

o

of some irrelevant detail, such as objects of similar colour. They have acknowledged the relevance of these disturbances in perceptual activity to the learning process:

> If the cerebral palsied child has handicaps in the sensory and perceptual fields or is mentally retarded it would appear naturally to follow that he would have handicaps in the more advanced stages of thinking owing to retardation in the earlier stages of learning or to absence of basic skills, such as ability to perceive objects in correct relationship.

Tansley & Gulliford (1962), working with mentally retarded children at a residential E.S.N. school, have drawn similar conclusions. They reported that many of the children were slower to classify and to see which things belonged together, and had difficulty in appreciating how known facts could be applied to new situations. They concluded that this was responsible for the fact that the children were seen to be 'poor at problem solving, comprehension work, and making generalisations'.

Wolff (1946) has been reported by Caldwell (1956) to have described this difficulty as a confusion in concept formation in which, 'the facts he knows are isolated facts, not organised as to their proper content'. This characteristic is symbolic of what Cruickshank & Raus (1955) have called 'Dissociation'. They explained:

> The individual has difficulty in relating parts to the total configuration. The greater tendency is towards segmentation of the whole with the ultimate possibility that the whole or gestalt is never perceived by the subject.

This represents the inability of some children to organise various aspects of a situation into significant and coordinated groups. It is a perceptual disability that can be seen in the performance of some children in tests such as the 'Block Design' (Wechsler, 1949). When they attempt to assemble the test material into a given pattern they often achieve groupings which are haphazard and meaningless.

In order to reduce the learning problems caused by disturbances in perception, several programmes for remedial perceptual training have been devised.

Gallagher (1960) was concerned with the confusion caused

by disturbances in figure-ground relationships. He used some of the methods and techniques that had been developed by Strauss & Lehtinen (1948). They included materials that exaggerated the important cues in order to facilitate the perceptual process of structuring and organising sensory impressions. For example, letters, which appeared in large print on plain contrasting backgrounds, were delineated with colour cues and with paper placed between the words to make them more easily distinguishable. A child was taught to lip read by a teacher who used an excessive amount of lipstick to provide a more obvious cue. Lessons included such activity as cutting, sorting, and manipulating objects with the use of self-instructive materials that necessitated only a minimum of assistance from the teacher. Gallagher (1964) reported, however, that experimental evaluation of this type of training programme for brain injured children had been scarce. Many difficulties were seen to exist in recognising and catering for the tremendous range of differences among children who were labelled 'brain injured'.

The Frostig Approach

Frostig & Horne (1964) have attributed many of the learning difficulties of children, particularly in respect of their reading and writing skills, to defects or a developmental lag in certain abilities involved in visual-perception. They have reported:

> Our research indicates that children who score low in tests of visual-perception are frequently lowest in academic achievement and most poorly adjusted in the classroom.

They have further suggested that as many as 25% of the children entering first grade have not reached the stage of 'perceptual maturity' that is necessary for them to be able to cope satisfactorily with their first lessons in reading, writing and arithmetic.

Many of the learning problems arising from visual-perceptual disabilities have been associated with the difficulties that a child may have in recognising objects and their relationships to each other. The effect that this deficit has upon a child's motor responses has been described by Frostig & Horne (1964) in the following terms:

> Since his world is perceived in a distorted fashion, it appears to him unstable and unpredictable. He is likely to be clumsy

in his performance of everyday tasks and inept at sports and games.

Such a diagnosis does not exlude the possibility of other causal effects. Although Frostig has directed her approach to 'training the lagging areas of perceptual development' she would, no doubt, agree with Tansley (1968) and others who have remarked upon the difficulty of differentiating between developmental lags and possible neural dysfunction. Irrespective of the causes, however, Tansley has advocated the use of structured programmes of perceptual training for the 'vast majority of neurologically abnormal children' who 'have perceptual handicap'. Tansley's concern for the various conditions of neurological abnormalities, in addition to perceptual and language problems, is the basis of his *remedial* approach to the training of children in E.S.N. and Special Schools. The programmes of movement and perceptual training that he has devised, in contrast with Frostig's 'psycho-educational methods', are therefore more closely linked with the medical rather than the psychological diagnoses of the children's learning problems.

Training exercises in visual perception form an important part of the Frostig programme of 'diagnostic' or 'clinical teaching'. The effectiveness of her approach is largely dependent upon the validity of the diagnostic procedures that she has employed and the ability of the teacher to translate the test results into efficient remedial programmes. These are concerned with the total development of the child and planned to rectify any imbalance in the areas of sensory-motor development, language, perception, social and emotional development and the development of the 'higher thought processes' of abstract thinking and concept formation.

Frostig has identified these areas to represent the various stages of a child's growth and development during which the emergence and training of certain abilities are particularly important.

The maximal development of a child's sensory-motor functions during the first two years of his life arises out of his exploration and a growing awareness of himself and his immediate environment. Plessey & Kuhlen (1957) describe this period for the child as being, 'devoted to the fascinating but difficult problem of getting control of its own body'. Isaacs

(1960) sees it as the time when the child 'constructs in his mind a basic working model of the world which he can use for the assimilation of experience'.

Following this phase of increased sensory-motor development is the period of rapid development of language.

> The child uses language to label and thus stabilise his world. He uses it to reinforce his actions and also as a means of communicating his needs and feelings to others.
>
> (Arkwright, 1969)

The development of a child's perceptual functions is very much dependent upon the successful training of the abilities that have emerged during these previous phases. By the same token, a child's progress into the higher realms of reasoning and abstract thinking is largely determined by the adequacy of his sensory-motor and language experiences.

In an attempt to identify the strengths and weaknesses of a child's sensory-motor functions, Frostig has proposed that an assessment be made and training directed where necessary to the following aspects of motor performance:

(i) flexibility
(ii) strength
(iii) speed and agility
(iv) balance
(v) rhythm
(vi) gross and fine motor coordination
(vii) laterality of eye, hand and foot
(viii) eye movements.

According to the child's capabilities in these areas, varying emphasis is placed upon each of the following aspects of a programme of physical education which is integrated with perceptual training and other programmes.

Training in whole-body coordination

This is introduced with a variety of simple locomotor activities (that have been suggested by Cratty) including crawling, skipping, balancing, and some imaginative games, which are intended to enhance control of the body as a prerequisite of the more advanced agility movements through which a child's strength and flexibility are developed.

In his own programme of physical activities Cratty (1969) has included only a very limited amount of formal training in strength, flexibility and cardiovascular endurance. This is in accordance with the major emphasis that he places upon the acquisition of physical recreational skills as a more effective means of ensuring the development of these qualities. He states:

> I believe that an increased tendency to participate in vigorous activities comes about when the child perceives he is becoming more competent in the skills required.

It would appear that Kephart holds a similar view in respect of physical fitness training. Although he has included the Kraus–Weber Tests (1954) as a *measure* of minimum muscular fitness he makes no direct reference to the specific development of these physical attributes.

Training in fine-motor coordination

This is centred upon simple hand-eye coordination skills such as tracing, cutting, pasting, and model making. These kindergarten activities are intended to provide a useful foundation for the introduction of the more complex hand-eye coordination skills such as catching and aiming a ball, and the important skills involved in the everyday activities of tying-up shoe laces and ribbons, and using simple tools, etc.

The development of body awareness

Frostig & Horne (1964) have stressed the need for the child to develop an adequate knowledge of his own body as the basis for the accurate perception and location of objects in his visual field. She describes 'an adequate knowledge of the body' in terms of the following three constituent elements:

(a) Body Image: referred to as the 'subjective experience' or 'feeling' that a child has of his own body, derived from internal sensory stimuli and from the impressions he has gained of the reactions of other people.
(b) Body concept: described as the knowledge that a child has of his body and of the functions of the different parts.
(c) Body schema: regarded as the unconscious self adjusting mechanisms of the body which coordinate movements and maintain equilibrium according to the changing positions of the body and the constant inflow of sensory information.

An example of the so called 'physical exercises' that have been used to develop the sense of body awareness are described by Jakeman (1967) in her report of some of the remedial work at the Franklin Delano Roosevelt School in London.

They learned to conquer space by climbing ladders, using balance boards, crawling through tunnels, and then learned to recognise the positions of their bodies in relation to objects, climbing *on* a chair, *over* a block, *under* a table, *in* a box, *out* of a circle, etc., and always the activity was reinforced with verbalisation.

It is interesting to compare this approach with the more direct method that Cratty (1969) has employed to encourage the child to form an accurate assessment of his own movement capabilities. This involves the child in an evaluation of his *actual* performances on *specific* tasks in terms of his *expected* performances. Cratty has made the point that children who lack the success of their peers tend, from feelings of inferiority, to under-estimate their own capabilities. By this measure (which Cratty has referred to as 'the evaluation of a child's concept of his performing self') a child may become more aware, not only of the standard of his performance but of any improvements that future practice may bring.

Eye-movement exercises

These are included as a supplement to the paper and pencil exercises that form the bulk of the training in visual-perception. They represent an attempt to develop a child's ability to direct and control his eye movements in focusing and following moving objects, and to stimulate his peripheral vision.

This physical education programme is intended not only to counteract any lag in a child's sensory-motor development but also to provide him with a rich and varied movement experience as a foundation for his training in visual perception. Until quite recently, however, Frostig (1968) appeared to hold certain reservations with regard to the value of a pure movement approach to the child's physical education:

Unfortunately the recognition of the importance of movement for development has sometimes led to over-emphasis, with movement education being made the basis of all other educational measures. This practice can be dangerous for it sometimes leads to unnecessary neglect or harmful postponement of other important educational goals.

Although Frostig acknowledged the 'great importance for all children' of movement education, 'especially for those with motor defects', she devoted relatively little attention to the indirect teaching method and creative aspects of this work. Her new movement education programme, as its title, 'Move, Grow, Learn' indicates, represents a slight shift of emphasis towards a broader *educational* approach to the development of the physical, creative and perceptual aspects of a child's total development. Nevertheless, the direct method of teaching set movement patterns is still very much in evidence and the stated aims of the programme which include the development of 'awareness of time and space, the ability to solve problems, and the ability to learn' must be viewed with a certain amount of speculation.

Frostig's most important contribution to the education of children with learning difficulties has been in the means that she has provided for the evaluation and training of deficits in a child's visual-perceptual abilities. For each of the five areas covered by the Developmental Test of Visual Perception, Frostig has provided training exercises in the form of work books and recommendations for more dynamic forms of sensory-motor training by way of physical exercises and work with three-dimensional objects.

Training in eye-motor coordination intends not only to increase a child's vocabulary of motor skills but also to enhance his understanding of the environment and develop a more sophisticated awareness of his own body and its capabilities. The work book exercises, as a follow-up from those in the visual-perceptual test provide a form of programmed learning through a series of progressively difficult exercises. These involve drawing, colouring and tracing lines between increasingly narrow boundaries until the child is able to orientate his drawing independent of any guide lines. As a preparation for these simple hand-eye coordination skills, Frostig has suggested work with a variety of different pieces of small apparatus including peg and marble boards, wooden blocks and beads, etc., in order to develop a child's kinesthetic and tactile perceptual abilities. These are believed to play an important part in his learning of the fine manipulative skills of handwriting, cutting, model making, drawing, and other kindergarten activities. In pursuit of similar objectives with hand-eye coordination exercises Cratty (1969) has emphasised the need to develop 'flexibility' through the use of a variety of drawing tasks and materials. He speaks of such development in terms of a child 'who can write on a variety of writing surfaces in a number of planes, and one who can execute a number of types of movements in all directions relative to his body'.

In her attempt to provide a wider range of experiences in visual-motor coordination, Frostig has also drawn attention to the need for 'a well balanced physical education programme' incorporating the active use of the whole body. Based on the supposition that, 'for many children, large movements are a necessary preliminary to the fine motor movements required in writing and similar activities', the programme both precedes and supplements the sheet exercises. It is aimed at developing a child's strength and flexibility in the trunk and lower limbs as part of his training in gross motor skills, such as running, jumping, climbing, and skipping, etc. Visual-motor skills training with the use of small apparatus such as balls, hoops and bean-bags, etc., is included to develop the skills necessary for the child to achieve not only the success that he seeks in games but also the coordination of vision and movement of the limbs that underly the whole-body skills of everyday living.

Training in figure-ground perception is aimed at improving a child's ability to select and focus his attention upon the relevant stimuli in his visual field and to ignore the irrelevant stimuli. It is also intended to increase the efficiency with which a child scans the display and his ability to shift his attention as the situation changes.

The paper and pencil exercises in figure-ground perception (Workbook II) approach the task of discriminating between complex overlapping and hidden figures by progressive practices of tracing intersecting lines and by outlining and colouring simple geometric shapes and figure drawings. To run concurrently with this work, Frostig has suggested exercises involving three-dimensional objects. The lesson may therefore include such activities as identifying and sorting objects from a large box into various categories according to their size, colour or shape characteristics. The children may be encouraged to shift their attention by picking out and naming different objects from a collection, or by pointing to certain objects in the classroom that the teacher asks them to identify.

In order to facilitate his concentration in reading, for example, a child may be encouraged to use a template through which he can see only one word or letter at any time. This effectively covers up the other words that may distract his attention. By using a ruler or by following the words with his finger a similar effect can be obtained. Working on the same principle the teacher may decide to reduce the number of over-all distractions that compete for the child's attention in the normal classroom situation. By removing pictures, eliminating excessive noise and movement, and by working for short periods within a clearly structured routine, a child may be encouraged to direct more of his attention to the stimuli that are relevant to the task in hand.

Training in form perception aims at increasing the child's ability to recognise objects irrespective of their size, colour or position. The Workbook (III) deals with the perceptual *constancies* of such qualities as shape, hue and colour. The training of a child to recognise certain categories of shapes regardless of other qualities is introduced through simple exercises in matching and in the identification of common objects and geometric forms, such as circles and rectangles, that may be presented in different colours and on differently structured backgrounds. Training in size constancy is very much dependent upon a child's familiarity with the actual objects themselves, for he is asked to recognise and compare the size differences of real objects and, on the basis of these experiences, to recognise such similarities between pictures of objects presented at different angles. The workbook exercises are therefore preceded by a considerable amount of practical work in manipulating objects of different shapes and sizes, in colouring, matching, and sorting them according to various categories.

Training in the perception of position in space is fundamentally linked with the development of an awareness of the body as a point of reference from which objects are located. Through an understanding of the coordinates of 'left', 'right', 'front' and 'behind', etc., in relation to different parts and positions of his own body a child may learn to associate and apply such directional terms in the location of the objects that he sees around him. In order to promote this sense of body awareness Workbook IV deals initially with the subject of reversals and rotations in exercises that require the children to identify from a series of pictures, those which occupy the same positions as the stimulus figures. Following on from this they may be asked to observe and discriminate between the left and right sides of the children in the pictures and then to adopt the same body positions themselves, and to touch and move their arms and legs following verbal directions and demonstrations by the teacher. A later progression from this includes exercises in drawing the mirror image of given patterns by filling in a number of squares on a large grid. Of perhaps greater value than the paper and pencil type exercises for the development of a more sophisticated body concept are the experiences that a child may obtain by using his whole body to explore the movement possibilities in situations involving large and small apparatus. Either by following verbal instructions such as finding different ways of getting over, under and round the apparatus, or by freely using the apparatus to experiment with the fundamental movements of, for example, climbing *up* the ladder, walking *along* the beam, or crawling *through* the hoops, a child may learn to understand the meaning of these terms through his actual physical experiences of them.

Training in the perception of spatial relations is a direct progression of the work of locating the position of objects in relation to the various coordinates of the body. It aims to develop the ability to perceive objects, or parts of a total configuration, in relation to each other. In the initial learning stages, the constituent parts of a complex figure are individually perceived and systematically integrated to complete the whole picture. In practice, therefore, exercises in assembling models and jigsaw puzzles, and in copying patterns on peg and marble boards or following instructions in placing objects in certain positions in relation to each other have been used as an introduction to the Workbook exercises. These call for the identification of the positional relationships of objects and the completion of figure drawings. This is followed by activities which deal more specifically with the concept of progression and serial order. They include exercises similar to the Picture Arrangement and Object Assembly subtests of the W.I.S.C. together with practice in simple maze tracing and stringing beads together in a prescribed order.

Frostig has recommended that the use of the five Workbooks should run concurrently and be preceded by practical exercises with three-dimensional objects. The whole subject of visual perception training is therefore inextricably linked with kinesthetic, tactile, and auditory sense experiences that serve to reinforce the visual motor training.

Frostig (1968) has recognised the value of this aspect of the practical work:

> A child who is deficient in kinesthetic and tactile sensitivity will be clumsy and awkward and inefficient in his movements and impaired in getting acquainted with and handling the world of objects. Such a child may need both kinesthetic stimulation, which originates in movement, and tactile stimulation, through touching and being touched.

This view has also been expressed by Ayres (1963) who provisionally identified deficiencies in tactile functions as a basic factor in 'developmental apraxia' (a disability from which a child 'has difficulty directing his hands or his body in performing skilled or unfamiliar motor tasks'). In identifying a syndrome of dysfunction in form perception and the perception of position in space, Ayres has indicated the major part played by both the tactile and kinesthetic sense modalities. Her recognition of the value of training in these areas to meet such deficiencies which affect perceptual-motor functions adds support to Frostig's recommendations. Although this view is perhaps the most common, some educationalists have placed very little emphasis upon kinesthetic sense training. Espenschade (1958) represents this section of opinion by her following comments:

> These sensations make little appeal to the consciousness and at best they tend to be vague and lack precision. Sufficient information to provide a clear concept of the task rather than any awareness of 'feel' seems to determine the result of the task.

The concept of readiness

The growing interest of many educationalists in theories regarding the ontogeny of perceptual-motor abilities has led to a method of compensatory education for children with learning difficulties based upon the recapitulation of developmental sequences. Frostig (1964) speaks of 'training the lagging areas' of perceptual development, and Cruickshank *et al.* (1961) referred to the need to 'fill in the gaps' of a child's vocabulary of experiences. Tansley & Gulliford (1962) believe that, 'teaching must be planned so as to anticipate and prepare for the next stage of development', and Kephart (1960) attempts to 'get the child back on the track' by directing attention to the stage in development at which training failed.

Sutphin (1964), in her recommendations for the teaching of first grade children, describes her approach as 'Learning to Learn'. Her basic aim is to provide for 'a more effective foundation for all future learning' by a programme of 'directed development and perception'.

The basis of this type of approach is a general acceptance of the hypothesis that during the various stages of a child's development there are critical periods for learning. These are characterised by the individual's maximal susceptibility to particular types of stimulation. During these periods certain abilities are developed and specific skills are acquired which have a direct influence upon his future behaviour. Ausubel (1967) has described the learning during these brief periods of ontogeny in terms of 'actualising potential capabilities or developing in new directions'. Implicit in this belief is the corollary that a child, deprived of the necessary stimulation during a critical learning period, will suffer some permanent degree of retardation. This, however, is an extreme point of view for it is commonly believed that at a later stage many children are able to draw upon the transferable elements of a greater wealth of experience to enable them to learn the skills that they may have missed. It would be more accurate therefore to regard these children as suffering from the cumulative effects of a deficit which may inhibit future learning.

Typical of this approach are the ideas of Kamii & Radin (1967) which stem from Piaget's concepts of child development (Piaget, 1950). Their proposals for pre-school training are based upon a general recognition of the research findings of Sigel *et al.* (1965) and other workers who have studied the educational progress of 'underprivileged' children. They put forward the idea that pre-schools designed to compensate for inadequate development should build for the future development of the child by recapitulating the sensory-motor stages of development (which Piaget has attributed to the first two years of life) and then progress through each succeeding stage ensuring that none are omitted.

Both Frostig (1968) and Kephart (1960) also identified the various stages of a child's development and produced batteries of tests that purport to assess the levels of development that the child has reached. An indication of the area and extent to which training is needed is provided by comparing a child's performances on the tests with the norms that have been obtained for children of the same age.

The validity of this system of screening is very much dependent upon the hypothesis that there are distinct abilities involved in the more complex perceptual-motor skills. In addition it is assumed that a child must have reached a certain level of development in these abilities as an essential requirement for his future progress. In accordance with this belief, several programmes of compensatory education have been devised for nursery and first grade children, with the expressed aim of preparing them for their future education at school. This approach assumes a knowledge not only of the precise nature of these basic abilities and of their development, but also of the way in which they are related to the learning of certain skills.

These basic levels of ability, assumed to be present in a 'normal' child, provide the starting point on which the school curriculum is based. However, the fact that there are certain relatively simple skills that a child may be unable to perform indicates that a wide discrepancy undoubtedly exists in these basic levels of ability. Gallagher (1966) described this as a 'developmental imbalance'. To account for this discrepancy Wedell (1968) has suggested that a child may have 'failed to develop some of the basic perceptual and cognitive skills on which learning, and particularly school learning is based'. He also added the reminder that these readiness skills can be selectively impaired.

The Kephart Approach
In accordance with this view Kephart (1960) identifies the child with potential learning problems as one who enters

school, 'with a lesser degree of skill and ability in one or more areas than the educational curriculum assumes'. He therefore calls for a reappraisal of the activities and teaching techniques at first grade level in favour of a more viable approach which is adaptable to the needs of the children. Accordingly, he has attempted a break-down of the basic skills into more simplified preparatory activities with the aim of avoiding some of the difficulties that children have in learning complex skills. Kephart (1968) has summarised the main objectives of his work as follows:

> . . . to identify some of these more basic skills, to suggest methods by which deficiencies in these skills can be detected, and to suggest training procedures which will attack the basic skills more directly.

In pursuit of the first of these objectives Kephart stresses the importance of early movement experience and movement training as the bases for perceptual development and future success in learning perceptual-motor skills. His approach is concerned not so much with training in specific skills as with the more generalised activities, and in particular, those related to the development of body image, lateral and directional awareness, and the perceptual abilities of spatial and form discrimination.

The development of body image as a frame of reference for the location of objects and the discrimination of their spatial relationships is described by Kephart (1960) as a 'learned concept'. The growing awareness that a child has of his own body develops from an increasing wealth of sensory impressions and experiences of movement. He learns to identify the different parts of his body and their relationship to each other and to external objects by experimenting with movements and later verbalising them in positional and directional terms. The spatial concepts, such as 'left', 'right', 'up', and 'down', acquire meaning and significance through his visual and kinesthetic impressions of the different movements. It is Kephart's view that a child learns to adjust and respond more purposefully to the world around him as a result of this increased positional and directional awareness.

The development of laterality and directionality. Progress towards greater differentiation within the body concept and function begins with the learned ability to discriminate between the left and right sides of the body. Kephart believes that the bilaterally symmetrical placement of the limbs and of the sense receptors and nerve pathways plays a significant part in this process. This provides two relatively independent 'sources' of sensory impressions from which the child can learn to distinguish between the two sides of the body. This discrimination is facilitated as he establishes a preference to use a particular hand and foot. With the development of laterality a child begins to apply his learned concepts of 'right' and 'left' in the location of near objects. The progression here is by no means automatic, for as Kephart has pointed out, the learning of directionality is preceded by the complex process of learning to integrate the visual information of external objects with the established kinesthetic awareness on which the child has built his concept of laterality.

By experimenting with movements which he knows to be those of the right hand, for example, he may point to or touch an object which then becomes a part of his concept of 'right'. These directional concepts are projected into the world around him as his awareness of the coordinates of his own body leads him to identify the same coordinates of space. Kephart (1960) has explained:

> He learns to translate the right-left discrimination within himself into a right-left discrimination among objects outside himself.

From the 'egocentric localisation' of objects the development of spatial relationships progresses with the ability to locate objects in relation to each other (i.e. 'objective localisation').

The ability to perceive spatial relationships is developed from an awareness of the location of objects in relation to the body. Kephart describes how a child first estimates the distance of an object in terms of the movement required for him to reach it (i.e. 'the translation of movement into space'). From his ability to locate objects in space a child learns to locate them in relation to each other. He refers to this, 'stabilising of the space world', as one of the most complicated readiness skills.

The development of form perception is described by Kephart in terms consistent with the theory of progress towards greater differentiation of the individual elements that constitute a child's total impressions of his external world. He has suggested that from this 'ill-defined mass' which Werner (1948) has called 'globular form', a child learns to identify the single elements that characterise a particular form. This process of learning to differentiate the qualities of various forms extends over many years. A child learns to perceive not only the separate details of a particular form but also the way in which these are combined to give the form a unique character with new and individual qualities of its own. Strauss & Kephart (1955) refer to this as 'constructed form' which is defined as, 'the organisation of the details previously differentiated out of the globular form into an integrated, coordinated unit' (Kephart, 1960). This ability of a child to organise his impressions into meaningful 'units' provides him with the means of dealing with the wealth of sensory information that is avilable to him at any one time.

From the development of these abilities emerge the readiness skills that are considered to be important in future learning. As Kephart has illustrated, many of the learning difficulties that a child may encounter at school appear as a direct result of a breakdown in the development of these abilities. In order to identify the point at which the breakdown may have occurred he has devised a 'Perceptual Survey Rating Scale'. Unlike the customary form of achievement tests with their standardised systems of scoring, Kephart has provided a series of graded tasks designed to permit *observation* of a child's perceptual-motor performances at the various developmental levels. With each task he has included his own observations to assist the teacher in his assessment of the adequacy of a child's responses, and in the identification of the areas of weakness and level of perceptual-motor development. The training is basically aimed at strengthening these weaknesses as they appear in the following broad areas of development: Sensory-motor learning, ocular control, and form perception.

Sensory-motor training is centred on a number of set activities and games involving a relatively few pieces of apparatus.

(*a*) The Walking Board provides for a number of balancing movements with progressions in walking backwards and side-

P

ways, in turning and balancing. Experience of these movements are intended to contribute to a greater kinesthetic awareness of the lateral postural adjustments required to maintain the body in a balanced position.

(*b*) The Balance Board enables the child to appreciate the effects that different movements have in changing the position of his Centre of Gravity.

(*c*) The Trampoline allows more freedom of movement as the body is momentarily released from the effects of gravity. The coordination required in maintaining the body in a balanced position is linked with an appreciation of the rhythm enduced by sequence work. From this, and from a child's own observations and kinesthetic sensations of his movements Kephart believes that he may also develop a greater awareness of the location and relationships of the different parts of his body.

In many of the set exercises that Kephart has devised for the Trampoline, and in recommending the use of certain percussion instruments he has been directly concerned with the development of the concept of rhythm. In part justification of this he has tenuously related the ability to establish and maintain rhythm patterns to the process by which serial information from individual sense modalities is kept classified and integrated in its correct temporal sequence. This theory also assumes that the perception of temporal relationships is part of the process by which the constituent elements of a given form are integrated.

With a slightly different view of the influence of a young child's concept of rhythm upon the process of integrating perceptual information, Sutphin (1964) has suggested that, '. . . this rhythm cancels out anything that is pending.' This refers to the unsolved problems and the information which the child, at that moment in time, has difficulty in integrating. Sutphin has associated a young child's sense of rhythm with the slow delta rhythm that predominates in his brain, and has hypothesised that by the 8th year when this has begun to change to an alpha rhythm, the child becomes more capable of sustaining his concentration.

This theory may explain the reference that Cratty (1969) has made to a child's 'natural preferences' to perform certain tasks such as tapping and walking with a *characteristic* rhythm (i.e. a 'personal tempo'). It may also account for the apparent difficulty that some children have in following certain rhythmic tempos.

Similar claims have been made for the use of eurythmics in the Rudolph Steiner schools. Geuter (1962) associates the Art of Eurythmy with the development of a child's powers of concentration and imitation, and speaks of the effect of, 'harmonising the bodily movements so that the skill to use the limbs and the different parts of the body develops'. de Havas, (1954) has described various planned exercises, in the Rudolph Steiner tradition, that are performed to music. The aim of this work which is described as training in the sense of movement, is to absorb the child's concentration in the feeling of the movements of the different parts of the body.

The fact that very little experimental evidence is available to support these hypothetical claims has not deterred the recent increase in the use of music and rhythm in programmes of compensatory education. It is difficult to measure such qualities as enjoyment, freedom, and creativeness in a child's responses, but many sensitive teachers are aware of the quality and range of movement that a child is capable of producing under the stimulus of music and rhythm.

Training in ocular control is primarily aimed at developing a child's ability to direct the movements of his eyes and maintain the focus on a given stimulus. Kephart regards this as a complex skill demanding a high degree of accuracy and precision. The learning of this is believed to be a vital factor in the subsequent development of directionality. The process is described by Kephart:

> When a child has learned this control, he matches the movement of his eyes to the movement of his hand and this transfers the directionality information from the kinesthetic pattern in his hand and arm to the kinesthetic pattern in his eye.

As a basis for the training in ocular control Kephart has devised a programme of set exercises which require the child to follow a moving target with his eyes. At different stages throughout the training the target is changed from a pencil to a pen-shaped electric torch (in order to increase the intensity of the visual stimulus) and then to a ball which is suspended on a piece of string. At a later stage the child is given the opportunity of matching the visual information with the kinesthetic impressions of pointing and then touching the target with his finger and hand. As the training proceeds the children are encouraged to work in pairs using similar pursuit-training activities and to progress to a wider range of activities including games, such as volley ball and basket ball. Many of these practices are similar to the eye-movement exercises that Frostig has used for stimulating peripheral vision and training in focusing and following regular and irregular movements of objects.

There can be few other educationalists, with the possible exception of Frostig, who have devoted so much attention to the training of the mechanisms that control the movements of the eyes. The noticeable absence of any such formal training from other programmes of compensatory education may be accounted for by the following possible explanations:

(*a*) It may be assumed that, in children of school age, the development of ocular control is already adequate for the visual-motor tasks that they are required to perform.

(*b*) Many educationalists may feel that the responsibility for identifying and correcting any defects in the visual mechanisms should remain in the hands of the ophthalmologist or school doctor. Most authorities, however, have acknowledged the value of close co-operation with the medical and other professions. Tansley & Gulliford (1960) in particular, have welcomed the general principle of corporate responsibility. They have also reminded us that:

> There are many children with visual defects which . . . cannot be confirmed without a neurological examination.

In his approach to training in ocular control, Kephart (1960) believes that:

> Most of the slow learning children who will be encountered in the classroom situation will evidence only minor difficulties revealed by slight irregularities in the ocular pursuit task.

Accordingly, he has directed his attention, not to the correction of any physical or major functional defects, but to the task of ensuring that the children are able to use their ocular mechanisms effectively.

(*c*) Educationalists may be satisfied that a programme of varied visual-motor activities already contains an adequate amount of exercise in ocular control.

The decision that many teachers have taken to exclude specific training in ocular control may be influenced by the lack of sufficient empirical evidence to support Kephart's belief in the positive transfer of effects to other areas of visual-motor learning. Cratty (1969) has commented on this point in his reference to the visual training that has been encouraged by the Optometric Extension Programme in America:

> It is surprising that, within the many years during which these practices have been engaged in, so few definitive studies have been produced attending to their worth.

Although there appears to be a general consensus of opinion that an improvement in ocular efficiency may resolve certain perceptual difficulties, particularly in respect of a child's reading problems, the manner in which such improvement can be most profitably effected must remain the subject of a certain amount of speculation.

Training in form perception, according to Kephart's approach, incorporates the use of set pieces of equipment including jigsaw puzzles, form and marble boards, match-stick figures, and peg boards. With this apparatus he has devised practical situations in which the perceptual processes of identifying, organising and integrating the various parts of a given object or figure is matched with the physical reality of actually performing this sequence of operations. By the same token, the pictures and other materials have been chosen for their relative simplicity of form and the ease with which they can be differentiated from their background. In manipulating or drawing the more complex figures, Kephart has proposed the use of a template which effectively blocks out all extraneous stimuli in the immediate visual field.

The recommended use of jigsaw puzzles and simple geometric shapes on the form board appear as an obvious choice of activities for training in constructive form perception. In these particular exercises the child is encouraged to 'integrate the constituent elements' on the basis of their perceived relationship to the total configuration.

In this work there is a considerable amount of overlap with Frostig's approach to the development of figure/ground discrimination and the perception of spatial relations. She has also made use of this type of apparatus in copying and matching exercises with puzzles, peg and marble boards. The value of these activities have also been appreciated by Cruickshank who has included several in his programme of hand/eye coordination exercises.

With the aim of providing a more viable form of training without the restrictions imposed by set exercises, both Kephart (1960) and Sutphin (1964) have demonstrated the possibilities that the use of the blackboard provides for freedom of expression and experimentation. Many children of school age who have not developed the precision and control required for the fine hand/eye coordination skills of pencil and paper work have improved as a result of this practice. Added to this is the opportunity for both the teacher and the child to observe the visual record of the traces of the movements. A child's observation of what represents a complete picture of his thoughts and expressions over a period of time is to him a continual source of fascination and incentive for this type of work.

Evaluation studies

From the very few studies that have attempted a comparison between different types of programmes there appears to be a good deal of conflicting evidence of their respective merits. Cratty (1969) reported that he could find no well-controlled research which could support any claims of either specific or general benefits for children with movement problems from the use of Kephart's perceptual-motor training. On the other hand, Brown (1968) and O'Connor (1969) have attributed improvements in certain measures of perception and motor ability to the effects of this programme. O'Connor referred to a study by Haring & Stables (1966) who obtained a significant improvement ($P<0.01$) in the performances of their Experimental Group of educable motor retardates on tests of Visual Perception and Eye-hand Coordination, after receiving Kephart's motor training programme. O'Connor also mentioned a study by Rutherford (1964) which included an evaluation of Kephart's approach in terms of the scores of two groups of 'normal kindergarten children', on the Metropolitan Readiness Test. It was reported that after a period of 11 weeks of 'free play combined with Kephart-orientated (1960) physical activity programme' the Experimental Group registered a significant improvement ($P < 0 \cdot 01$) over the group who participated only in the free play.

In her own study, O'Connor (1969) used a traditional physical education programme (which included 'elementary games, relays, calisthenics and folk dance') to compare with Kephart's programme of physical activities. The effects of these upon the performances of two groups of first grade children were recorded on tests of motor ability (i.e. Brace/Johnson test, 1942), perception (i.e. Perceptual Forms Test, Kephart, 1960) and academic achievement (i.e. Metropolitan Achievement Test). After a period of 6 months' training the retest scores indicated that the Experimental Group who had received the Kephart-type activities achieved a greater improvement on more than three-quarters of the motor ability items. With the exception of the scores on grip strength, all significant differences favoured the Experimental Group at the $0 \cdot 05$ level. On the Perceptual Forms Test and on both the Metropolitan Achievement and Readiness Tests, however, there were no significant differences between the performances of the two groups. From these results it was concluded that:

> The Kephart Programme appears to have merit for the elementary school physical education curriculum as children did improve.

The improvements in gross motor ability, however, were not seen to effect any changes in the perceptual or academic abilities of these first grade children.

Direct and indirect teaching methods

With the ready access that most teachers have to a selection of interesting pieces of apparatus, many of the activities suggested by Frostig and Kephart may be supplemented to provide more opportunities for experimentation and experiences of a wider range of movements. This possible extension of the programme would counteract the tendency of the children to learn the isolated skills involved in the set exercises. It would also support Kephart's expressed aim of 'helping the children to generalise rather than merely to acquire a specific skill'. The theme of freedom for experimentation is the essence of the physical education programme recommended by Tansley & Gulliford (1960). They have included a wide range of both large and small pieces of apparatus with the aim of encouraging the children, 'to use their natural activity, e.g. climbing, walking, running, skipping, catching, throwing'. In these periods which are referred to as free physical activity lessons, they have observed the children increase in 'confidence, initiative and co-operativeness'. By indirect teaching methods the children are encouraged to create their own movement patterns according to their individual aptitudes and abilities.

In contrast to this approach, the direct method of teaching that Kephart and many others have employed encourages the learning of more stereotyped movement patterns. Kephart justifies this as an initial approach on the following grounds:

> From his education he has learned to make adaptions which have now become fixed and the inhibiting type of experimenting which the normal child uses to develop his higher degrees of skill becomes impossible for the slow learning child.

Without committing himself entirely to this approach Cratty frequently advocates a very direct teaching method. His explanation of this is partly expressed in his opinion that:

> The initial elimination of errors is better than attempting to later correct an 'ingrained' mistake.

Cratty has taken this a step further by including the teaching of standard procedures (i.e. 'work methods') for carrying out novel tasks. This he suggests is most important during the initial stages of learning, for a child's future success or failure in a particular task is very much determined by the effectiveness of the strategy that he has adopted. As an example Cratty (1969) has stated:

> He needs information how to arrange himself relative to the task, how to lay out materials, what to pick up first, and exactly how to hold an object in a construction task.

A form of compromise between these two methods appears to be the approach that has been adopted by the Cheshire Education Committee in their programme of physical education for retarded children:

> All children like to be successful and the regular practice of a movement often results in success. It is a discreet mixture of

challenge and accomplishment which produces the most satisfactory result.

The main advantages of providing the child with opportunities for experimenting with a wide range of movements lies with the assurance that what he learns is more likely to be transferrable to other situations. Cratty is particularly keen to ensure this positive transfer of learning, which he observes has a greater chance of occurring if several training tasks are employed in the learning of a skill. Referring to the stereotyping effects of repeated practice in isolated tasks he cites the example of a group of children who, after showing their proficiency in left-right discriminating movements in the 'Angels-in-the-Snow' game were unable to make similar judgements of laterality when they changed their body positions.

Cratty recommends the more positive approach of 'teaching for transfer' to encourage the maximum transfer of learning from one activity to another. This basically involves the application of some of the well-known theories which describe the conditions under which positive transfer is most likely to occur. He records the advantage of employing a *number* of activities which call for *similar* response elements, and the importance of explaining and demonstrating to the children not only the reasons why they are practising a particular skill but also the principles that underly the successful performance. For example, it is believed that a child may learn more easily how to balance on one foot if he *understands* that his body must remain in a position over the top of it.

Cratty would no doubt agree that many motor-impaired children, particularly those of lower intelligence, may have difficulty in understanding these principles. Burt (1957) has pointed out that:

> One striking difference between the dull child and the normal lies in the incapacity of the former to deal with abstract ideas and relationships.

This may partially account for the positive relationship that has been found to exist between intelligence and the rate of motor skills learning, within the range of subnormality. McCloy & Young (1954) have proposed an explanation for this which supports Cratty's view that the duller children are less capable of devising efficient work strategies and also have greater difficulty in transferring their previously learned material to a novel situation.

In recognising the limitations and the difficulties that a child may have in understanding the requirements of a given task, Oliver (1963) has adopted the principle of concentrating upon one objective at a time and of guiding the child in his learning through small progressive steps. This ensures that he understands how a movement is performed and is able to achieve a measure of success at each stage in learning the skill. In this approach each successive stage in the performance of a movement is clearly indicated to the child and, where necessary, his body is physically transported through the movement. Using auditory reinforcement the child is helped to initiate and sustain his movements by shouting and clapping the rhythm. The exaggeration of effort qualities such as quietness and loudness, lightness and heaviness, was also used with the observed effect of automatically correcting certain movements.

Oliver & Keogh (1967 and 1968), working with small groups of motor-impaired E.S.N. children both in England and in America, have had a considerable amount of success in using these methods in their physical education programmes. In respect of the content of their work, Oliver (1963) has outlined the activities that are appropriate for E.S.N. children at different age and ability levels. His belief in the theory of critical learning periods is reflected in the following comment:

> There is an optimum time in the child's physical development when conditions are most favourable for certain skills to be learned.

In the early school years, therefore, the accent is laid upon greater freedom of natural whole-body movements. The aim here is the development of body control and awareness through the provision of exploratory type activities using such small apparatus as bats, balls and hoops, etc. Also for this young age group Oliver (1955) advocates the teaching of the fundamental skills of throwing, kicking, catching, aiming and striking a ball. These he regards as being 'absolutely indispensable in the education of these children'. Priority has been given to this aim in order that the children may achieve success and self-confidence in their own ability to take part in the social games of their 'normal' peers. A similar approach has been put forward by Ablewhite (1961) who gives precedence to the teaching of the basic skills required in games over the development of skills required in other subjects.

In the secondary school years the activities that Oliver has recommended are more specialised and his approach is very much directed to the acquisition of recreational skills. This broader programme offers a wide range of challenging activities of high prestige and interest value, ranging from weight training and camping, to the competitive major games. The purpose of this programme is to search out and exploit the talents of each child. Burt (1957) explains this in the following terms:

> The duller child needs a sharper, a more varied, a more personal stimulus. . . . We must make the most of each child's strongest points and compensating abilities.

The task of developing a child's strengths and equipping him with the skills that will enable him to participate in some form of physical recreation has been treated by Oliver and other physical educationalists as a matter of some urgency. This has traditionally involved training in the prescribed patterns of movement that form the sensory-motor skills in such pursuits as swimming, athletics, olympic gymnastics and to a lesser extent those of the major team games.

The movement approach to compensatory education

In contrast to the teaching of these specific skilled movements a more indirect approach has accentuated the freedom of individual inventiveness and creative expression. By this means a child is relieved of the necessity to conform to set patterns of movement, and encouraged to create a wider and more meaningful vocabulary of movements. The work of the Reading Research Foundation of Chicago is an example of this type of approach which encourages the child with reading and movement problems to devise and control his own motor responses in a variety of challenging situations. Their movement programme which aims, 'to develop a state of readiness to learn', is based upon the Piagetian concept of developmental sequences:

> Piaget shows clearly how opportunity for variety in stimulation and response leads to cognitive growth, and how

behavioural exploration develops into curiosity. It is from this research tradition that we have devised the notion of avoiding the development of habits and skills in our exercise programme and, instead, have stressed the principle of continuously providing the child with some small increment of challenge.

From the work of Montessori, and her concept of human movement, in which the mind is seen to work and communicate through the body (i.e. 'realisation in action'), the idea of introducing the child to a vocabulary of movements and to an awareness of his movement capabilities became an accepted practice. Her view of education which accentuated the individualism of Rousseau and Frobel was motivated by her belief in the freedom and spontaneity of a child's development. She aimed to foster this spontaneity by recognising and training the basic abilities of the child. In reference to the Montessori method Argy (1965) states:

Her recognition that sensory organisation is dependent on the timing of cortical maturation and her method of directing activities of the child in a group situation seemed to offer an ideal method of correcting the defects that brain damaged children present.

Montessori's 'child-centred' approach was largely inspired by the work of Itard and Séguin. Itard applied Locke's thesis that the innate capacities of a child, given freedom of expression will emerge through his natural curiosity. Following on from Itard's emphasis on sense training, Séguin developed his 'physiological method'. This included systematic training of the senses and of the muscular and nervous systems by concentrating upon hand-eye coordination activities with pictures, coloured paper, scissors and modelling clay. Montessori elaborated upon this theme of 'sensationalism' by applying the sense training materials that she had previously used with mentally defective children to her work with children of normal intelligence.

Working on similar lines of informality and spontaneity through the medium of human movement, Sherbourne (1965) recognises the place of interest, physical needs, rhythm of effort and relaxation in her work with brain-damaged children. She stresses the need for the teacher to divorce himself from the formal and direct approach by working *with* the children, establishing a close personal relationship and winning their confidence. The use of music, rhythm and uninhibited movement are significant features of her work which embodies the realisation that 'movement is not just a physical activity, but an education of the person as an integral being—educating mental, intuitive, physical, emotional and social aspects'.

The possibilities of remedial programmes based upon music and movement as a medium of self-expression have been explored by a number of educationalists in recent years. Bruce (1969) recognises the creative art of movement as, 'the most fundamental of all languages'. She speaks of the sensitivity and absorbtion of E.S.N. children in movement and dance that compensates for the failure that they may have had in trying to learn some of the recognised motor skills. An interesting feature of this work is her appreciation of the different qualities that characterise the movements of individual children. She observes:

> These children, like any other people, have individual difficulties of extreme slowness or haste, heaviness, over-tension, or over-lightness, vagueness in the use of space, or an over-economic, erratic, or jerky gesture pattern. Their difficulties tend to be extreme.

This insight illustrates the opportunities that an observant teacher may have of identifying the deficiencies in a child's movements. The suggestions for 'individual movement therapy' put forward by Lamb (1953) rely upon this type of observation, 'to diagnose the strains in a person's movement'. On the basis of such analysis, rhythmic movement sequences have been devised to help the individual overcome his particular movement problems. The aim of this treatment as described by Lamb, is typical of this form of approach:

> The process compensates the lopsided, unbalanced factors, brings them into harmony simultaneously toning down exaggerated tendencies and building up neglected essentials.

Laban in his study of human movement was also concerned with the development and maintenance of this sense of proportion within the factors of motion. His view that,

Effort is transmitted more easily than thoughts, and economy of effort is the first pre-requisite of skill.

has prompted a close observation and awareness of movement from many sources. An article in the *Lancet* (1963) reports:

> In the organisation and development of skilled motor activity, there are many factors which are still obscure. As everyone knows, individuals vary in physical as in mental constitution. Whereas some are lithe and graceful in their movements, in others the coordination and control of muscular activity is much less efficient: movements often involve excessive expenditure of energy, with inaccurate judgement of the necessary force, tempo and amplitude. Such people are regarded as constitutionally clumsy.

Laban has proposed that all bodily actions may be assessed by means of effort elements and that a change of individual effort can be effected by appropriate training. On the basis of this assumption, Allen (1970) carried out a programme of effort analysis and training with a group of boys who were regarded as being motor impaired (i.e. their scores on Stott's test ranged between 11 and 22, with a mean of 15). These children, whose ages were between 8½ and 10 years, had IQ's ranging from 77 to 107, with an average of 92. At the time of the study they were attending a remedial centre, having been referred because of their backwardness in academic learning.

The purpose of the project was to attempt an assessment of the individual effort qualities in the movements of these children and to devise and carry out a programme of movement training aimed at correcting any noticeable deficiencies. The initial assessment of individual efforts was made by a small panel of independent experts who analysed films of the children's performances and a variety of selected activities. These items were chosen to cover a wide range of movements based upon the criterion of Stott's factors of motor performance. They included activities involving dynamic balance, hand-eye coordination, whole-body movements, manual dexterity, and simultaneous movements with both hands. Individual effort profiles were made in order to compare a child's responses with the effort components that the panel agreed upon in their analysis of each of these activities. The total number of incorrect responses was then calculated to give an indication of the area and extent to which training was needed.

On the basis of Laban's motion factors, his breakdown of the effort elements (each with two opposite components) were used in the movement analysis.

Table 12 gives an example of an individual profile showing the number of incorrect effort responses made by a child during his initial performances on the test battery:

TABLE 12

The EFFORT PROFILE of a boy aged 8 years

Laban's Motion Factors	Laban's Effort Elements	Number Incorrect Responses	% Incorrect Responses	RATING A–E	A 0–20	B 21–40	C 41–60	D 61–80	E 81–100
Weight	FIRM (16)	10	62·5	D					
	LIGHT (10)	3	30	B					
Time	SUDDEN (16)	4	25	B					
	SUSTAINED (10)	3	30	B					
Space	DIRECT (17)	10	58·8	C					
	FLEXIBLE (7)	2	28·6	B					
Flow	BOUND (18)	5	27·8	B					
	FREE (8)	0	0	A					

Total % Incorrect Responses 32·8
No. in brackets indicates possible correct responses.
MOST HELP NEEDED—FIRM, DIRECT.

(after Allen, 1970)

The twelve boys who took part in the study were divided equally into two matched groups according to their age and motor impairment score on Stott's test. The six who formed the Control Group received only their normal two periods of games each week. The Experimental Group received in addition, the following programme of movement training devised by

Allen & Morris (1970) for 2 × 40 minutes sessions per week over a period of seven weeks. In general terms, the programme aimed at developing in each child the ability to recognise, discriminate, express, and apply the different effort qualities in movement. The following synopsis represents an outline of the relevant features of the programme:

PHASE I. *Vocabulary building*

(*a*) Identification. Understanding of the individual effort qualities by seeing, hearing, saying and doing. Emphasis was placed on the elements which the child found the most difficult to reproduce.

(*b*) Discrimination between contrasting qualities. Learning to appreciate, verbally, visually and kinesthetically, the differences between, for example, a direct and a flexible movement.

(*c*) Conceptualisation. Learning to classify movements using similar effort qualities, e.g. quick running, quick rolling, quick eye and hand movements.

PHASE II. *Sequencing or sentence building*

(*a*) Sequences of activities and different qualities were given for each child to interpret according to his own capabilities, e.g. a strong jump followed by a sustained roll.

(*b*) (i) Individual experimentation of movement tasks. Simple sentences were built up by the children, using two or three different qualities.

(ii) Selection and repetition of sequences to show different degrees possible in the elements—very quick, very sustained, etc.

This was extended to cover a full range of basic actions, e.g. running, climbing, striking, balancing.

PHASE III. *Task orientation*

(*a*) Task analysis. The emphasis here was placed upon the *activities* which the child found the most difficult.

(*b*) Experimentation. Finding alternative ways of achieving the objective of the task, e.g. different ways of getting the ball into the basket, different ways of getting on and off a ledge.

(*c*) Analysis of individual responses in terms of the efficiency of the appropriate qualities involved in the selected movement.

(*d*) Selection and guidance practice of individual skill responses.

(*e*) Problem solving in a variety of skilled movement situations. e.g. catching, throwing, balancing.

In phases I and II, attention was focused upon the effort qualities and not primarily on the skill. In phase III, more emphasis was placed upon the skill, referring back to effort qualities. Both direct and indirect teaching methods were used throughout the three phases.

At the end of this training period both groups were re-tested on Stott's test.

From the re-test scores of the Experimental Group noticeable gains were recorded on all items, particularly on those representing dynamic balance. The fine manipulative movements required for the manual dexterity items which had presented the greatest difficulty to both groups appeared to be the least affected by the training programme.

In addition to any effects that the programme of movement training may have had to account for the greater improvement on all items of Stott's test by the Experimental Group, the fact that they received *extra* periods of physical education, irrespective of their content, no doubt also influenced these results. The relatively small number of children involved in the study prevents any firm conclusions from being drawn as to the value of this type of approach. These results, however, are sufficiently encouraging to support further investigations with this work.

References

Allen, W. (1970) An investigation into the motor impaired child with a view to devising a remedial programme based on Rudolf Laban's Principles of Movement. Unpublished essay. University of Leeds, Institute of Education.

Allen, W., Driver, P. J., Jones, J. C. & Mumtaz, A. (1970) Motor Impairment—Compensatory Education for the clumsy child. Unpublished dissertation. University of Leeds, Institute of Education.

Allen, W. & Morris, P. R. (1970)   A programme of movement training based on Laban's Principles of Movement. Unpublished paper. University of Leeds, Institute of Education.

Argy, W. P. (1965)   Montessori versus Orthodox. *Rehabilitation Literature*, 26: 10.

Arkwright, M. (1969)   *The Frostig Approach*. London: The College of Special Education.

Ausubel, D. P.   How reversible are the cognitive and maturational effects of cultural deprivation? In A. H. Passow, M. Goldberg & A. J. Tannenbaum (Eds.) (1967)   *Education of the disadvantaged*. New York: Holt, Rinehart & Winston.

Ayres, A. J. (1963)   The development of perceptual-motor abilities. A theoretical basis for treatment of dysfunction. The Eleanor Clarke Slagle Lecture. *Amer. J. of Occ. Therapy*, XVII, 6, 221–223.

Bender, A. L. (1945)   A visual motor gestalt test. *Research Monog. 3*. New York: Amer. Orthopsychiatric Assn.

Benton, A. L. (1945)   A visual retention test for clinical use. *Arch. Neurol. and Psychiat.*, 54, 212–216.

Brenner, M. W., Gillman, S., Zangwill, O. L. & Farrell, M. (1967)   Visuo-motor ability in school children. *Brit. Med. J.*, 4, 259–262.

Brown, R. C. (1968)   The effect of a perceptual-motor education program on perceptual-motor skills and reading readiness. Paper presented at the AAPHER Convention, St. Louis, April 1st.

Bruce, V. R. (1969)   *Awakening the Slower Mind*. London: Pergamon Press.

Burt, C. (1957)   *The Causes and Treatment of Backwardness*. London: University Press Ltd.

Carlwell, V. E. (1956)   *Cerebral Palsy, Advances in Understanding and Care*. New York: North River Press.

Cheshire Education Committee   *The Education of Dull Children at the Secondary Stage*. London: University Press, Ltd.

Cratty, B. J. (1969)   *Motor Activity and the Education of Retardates*. Philadelphia: Lea & Febiger.

Cruickshank, W. M. & Dolphin, J. E. (1951)   Educational implications of psychological studies of cerebral palsied children. *Except. children*, 18, 1–8.

Cruickshank, W. M. & Raus, G. M. (Eds.) (1955)   *Cerebral Palsy. Its Individual and Community Problems*. Syracuse: University Press.

Cruickshank, W. M., Bentzen, F. A., Ratzeburg, F. H. & Tannhauser, M. T. (1961)   *A Teaching method for brain injured and Hyperactive Children*. Syracuse: University Press.

de Havas, F. (1954)   Movement and rhythm in remedial education. *Mental Health*, 13, 2, 51–58.

de Havas, F. (1961)   Rudolf Steiner and Education. *The slow learning child*, 8, 68–73.

Espenschade, A. (1958)   Kinaesthetic awareness in motor learning. *Percept. & Motor Skills*, 8, 142.

Farnworth, M. (1970)   A consideration of reading readiness in terms of perceptual maturity. *Forward Trends*, Feb., 13–16.

Floyer, E. B. (1955) *A Psychological Study of a City's Cerebral Palsied Children*. London: Brit. Council for the Welfare of Spastics.
Francis-Williams, J. (1964) *Understanding and Helping the Distractible Child*. London: The Spastics Society.
Frostig, M., Lefever, W. & Whittlesey, J. R. B. (1963) *Developmental Test of Visual Perception*. Palo Alto: Consulting Psychologist Press.
Frostig, M. (1963) Visual perception of the brain injured child. *Amer. J. of Orthopsychiat*. 33, 665–671.
Frostig, M., Maslow, P., Lefever, D. W. & Whittlesey, J. F. C. (1964) *The Marianne Frostig Developmental Test of Visual Perception. 1963 Standardisation*. Palo Alto: Consulting Psychologists' Press.
Frostig, M. & Horne, D. (1964) *The Frostig Program for the Development of Visual Perception*. Chicago: Follet.
Frostig, M. (1966) *Developmental Test of Visual Perception—Administration and Scoring Manual*. Palo Alto: Consulting Psychologists' Press.
Frostig, M. (1968) Sensory-motor Development. *Special Education*, 57, 2, 18–20.
Gallagher, J. J. (1964) *The Tutoring of Brain Injured Mentally Retarded Children*. Illinois: Thomas.
Gesell, A. & Amatruda, C. S. (1941) *Developmental Diagnosis*. New York: Hoeber.
Geuter, I. (1962) *Adventure in Curative Education*. Netherlands: New Knowledge books.
Goldstein, K. (1936) The modification of behaviour consequent to cerebral lesions. *Psychiat. Quart*., 10, 568.
Hart, R. L. G. (1970) Perceptual deficiency. *Forward Trends*, Feb., 19–20.
Isaacs, J. (1960) *The Growth of Understanding in the Young Child*. London: Ward, Lock.
Jacobson, E. (1938) *Progressive Relaxation*. Chicago: University Press.
Jakeman, D. (1967) The Marianne Frostig approach. *Forward Trends*, 11, 3, 99–110.
Jakeman, D. (1968) Using the Frostig Programme. *Special Education*, June, 25–29.
Johnson, W. R. & Fretz, B. R. (1967) Changes in perceptual-motor skills after a children's physical developmental program. *Percept. & Motor Skills*, 24, 610.
Kamii, C. K. & Radin, N. L. (1967) A framework for a pre-school curriculum based on some Piagetian concepts. *J. of Creative Behaviour*, 1, 3, 314–323.
Kephart, N. C. (1960) *The Slow Learner in the Classroom*. Ohio: Merrill.
Laban, R. & Lawrence, F. C. (1947) *Effort*. London: MacDonald & Evans.
Laban, R. (1948) *Modern Educational Dance*. London: MacDonald & Evans.

Laban, R. (1960) *The Mastery of Movement.* 2nd Edition, revised by Ullmann, L. London: MacDonald & Evans.

Lamb, W. (1953) Individual movement therapy. *Mental Health*, 13, 15–19.

Lancet (1963) Clumsy children. *Lancet*, 1, 1252.

McCloy, C. H. & Young, M. D. (1953) *Tests and Measurements in Health and Physical Education.* New York: Appleton-Century Crofts.

Miller, E. & Rosenfeld, G. B. (1952) The psychological evaluation of children with cerebral palsy and its implications and treatment. *J. Pediatrics*, 41, 613–621.

O'Connor, C. (1969) Effects of selected physical activities upon motor performance, perceptual performance and academic achievement of first graders. *Percept. & Motor Skills*, 29, 703–709.

Oliver, J. N. (1955) Physical education for educationally subnormal children. *Educational Review.* 8, 122–136.

Oliver, J. N. (1963) The physical education of E.S.N. children. *Forward Trends*, 7, No. 3, 87–90.

Oliver, J. N. & Keogh, J. F. (1967) Helping the physically awkward. *Special Education*, 56, 22–26.

Oliver, J. N. & Keogh, J. F. (1968) A clinical study of physically awkward E.S.N. boys. *Res. Quart.*, 39, 301–307.

Pedder, R. A. (1964) Observations on distractibility. Oxford Study Group. Report to The Spastics Society, London.

Piaget, J. (1950) *The Psychology of Intelligence.* New York: Harcourt.

Plessey, S. L. & Kuhlen, R. G. (1957) *Psychological Development throughout the Life Span.* New York: Harper & Rowe.

The Reading Research foundation (1967) *Perceptual Motor Training.* Chicago: Illinois.

Schaffer, H. R. (1958) Objective observations of personality development in early infancy. *Brit. J. of Med. Psych.*, 31, 174.

Sherbourne, V. (1965) *Movement for Mentally Handicapped Children.* Bristol Dept. of Students of the National Association of Mental Health.

Signy, Q. G. E. (1960) Remedial work in the junior school. *Forward Trends*, 4, No. 4, 160–164.

Smith, D. W. & Smith, P. C. (1966) Developmental studies of spatial judgments by children and adults. *Percept. & Motor Skills*, 22, 3–73.

Strauss, A. A. & Werner, H. (1942) Disorders of conceptual thinking in brain injured children. *J. Nerv. Ment. Dis.*, 96, 153.

Strauss, A. A. & Lehtinen, L. C. (1948) *Psychopathology and Education of the Brain Injured Child.* New York: Grune & Stratton.

Strauss, A. A. & Kephart, N. C. (1955) *Psychopathology and Education of the Brain Injured Child.* New York: Grune & Stratton.

Sutphin, F. E. (1964) *A Perceptual Testing—Planning Handbook for First Grade Teachers.* U.S.A.: Boyd. Bros.

Talkington, L. W. (1968) Frostig visual perceptual training with low-ability-level retarded. *Percept. & Motor Skills*, 27, 505–506.

Tansley, A. E. (1960) The education of neurologically abnormal children. *Times Educat. Suppl.*, Jan. 20th.

Tansley, A. E. & Gulliford, R. (1960) *The Education of Slow Learning Children.* London: Routledge & Kegan Paul.

Tansley, A. E. (1968) Some aspects of the differential diagnosis and treatment of neurologically abnormal children. Paper read at Conference, Jan. 2nd. Published by the College of Special Education, London, W.1.

Tyson, M. C. (1963) Pilot study of remedial visuo-motor training. *Special Education*, LII, 4, 23–25.

Vernon, M. D. (1962) *The Psychology of Perception.* Harmondsworth: Penguin.

Wedell, K. (1964) *Some Aspects of Perceptual Motor Development in Young Children.* London: The Spastics Society.

Wedell, K. (1964) Perceptual-motor difficulties. *Special Education*, 54; 4, 25–30.

Werner, H. (1941) Psychological approaches investigating differences in learning distractibility. *Amer. J. of Ment. Def.*, 47, 269.

Werner, H. (1948) *Comparative Psychology of Mental Development.* New York: International Universities Press.

Wolff, W. (1946) *The Personality of the Pre-school Child.* New York: Grune & Stratton.

Author Index

Subject Index

Abdominal decompression, 42
Ability(ies), 29, 92, 93, 97, 104
  basic, 84, 86
  concept of, 83–88
  general, 83, 85
  hierarchy of, 87
  rhythmic, 161
  tactile perceptual, 217, 220
Ability-skill paradigm, 85
Abortion, 45
Activation, 30, 31, 62
Aetiology of motor impairment, 34,
  36–72
Affective development, 126
Age of readiness, 87
Agnosia, 56, 189
Albuminaria, 46
Alpha rhythm, 226,
Anaemia, 45, 48
Anaesthetics, 42, 51
Analysers, 29, 92, 93, 94
Angels-in-the-snow, 233
Anoxia, 41, 42, 43, 51, 105, 106
Antibodies, 44, 45
Apraxia, 56, 156, 189, 220
Approved school children, 185
Arthritis, 49
Arousal, 28, 29–31, 32, 63
Asphyxia, 51
Ataxia, 52, 54
Athetoid, 52
Attention, 25, 26, 32, 33, 94, 95, 127,
  130
  short-span, 156, 191, 202
  'switching' 130
Attraction response, 157
Autonomic nervous system, 29

Awkwardness, 113

Backwardness, 40
Balance, 80, 81, 225, 238, 241
  board, 226
Behaviour disorders, 41, 105
Binet intelligence scale, 160
Birth
  injury, 39, 42, 158
  premature, 42
  weight, 47
Blackboard, 230
Body
  awareness, 126, 127, 134
  boundary, 125
  concept, 123, 124, 127, 128, 130,
    132–136, 143, 214, 219
  consciousness, 134
  experience, 134
  image, 123, 124, 125, 127, 131,
    134, 136, 138–140, 141, 214,
    223, 224
  schema, 124, 131, 214
Bogardus fatigue test, 168
Brain, 21, 32, 39, 40, 43, 44, 45
  damage, 38, 41, 42, 55, 56, 66,
    82, 89, 105, 106, 110, 112, 115,
    118–120, 150, 153–158, 178, 180
  disorders, 52
  dysfunction, 41, 55–58
  injuries, 43, 158
  stem, 29, 30
Breech presentation, 49

Caesarian section, 51
Cell assemblies, 58, 75
Central mechanisms, 22, 24, 25, 26,
  29

Mumps, 44
Muscles, 21
Music, 227, 237

Nervous system, 23
Neural dysfunction, 55, 150, 156,
  158, 171, 180, 203, 212
  impairment, 115
  maturation, 95
Neuroticism, 118, 184
Non-dominant hemisphere, 157

Ocular, vacillation, 157
  control, 227, 228
Oestrogen, 46
Operant conditioning, 96
Optometric Extension Programme,
  229

Paediatrics, 10
Paraplegia, 55
Pelvic deformity, 49
Perception, 25, 26, 41, 93
  imposed-obtained, 64
  position in space, 192, 218, 219
  spatial relations, 192, 193, 219–
    220, 224, 229
  visual, 190–194, 208–212
Perceptual
  age, 193, 194
  deprivation, 56, 58, 59, 60, 64,
    109, 131
  learning, 96
  mechanisms, 108
  quotient, 193, 194
  speed, 97
  Survey Rating scale, 225
  systems, 22, 25, 26, 28, 33
Percussion instruments, 226
Peripheral vision, 228
Perseveration, 156, 190, 203, 204
Personality, 16, 118
  assessment, 183
Personal-social adjustment, 76
Physical education, 9, 140, 146
Pituitary, 47
Placenta, 43, 44, 45,
  praevia, 42, 48, 49, 51
Play, 137
Pneumonia, 44

Polio, 44, 49
Porteus Maze Test, 183
Pregnancy, 42, 44, 45, 47, 116, 117
Prematurity, 48, 49
Pre-programming, 25
Previous learning, 172
Progesterone, 46
Proprioception, 24, 25, 27, 29, 128,
  135
Psychiatric disorders, 159
Psychology
  developmental, 10
  gestalt, 208, 209
Psychophysical monism, 74
Pyramidal tract, 43, 157, 189

Quadriplegia, 55

Rail-walking Test, 170, 171
Reaction time, 78, 168, 183
Reactive inhibition, 118
Reading difficulties, 177, 191, 192,
  193, 211, 218
Re-education, 9
Respiration, 54
Reticular formation, 29, 30, 119
Rhesus
  incompatibility, 42
  factor, 45–46
Rheumatism, 53
Rhythm, 213, 226, 237
Rhythmic ability, 161
Rickets, 49
Rigidity, 54
Rubella, 44, 45
Rudolph Steiner schools, 227

Scarlet fever, 53
Schemata, 29, 75, 92, 94
Scoliosis, 49
Selective attention, 24, 26–27, 29, 64,
  65, 93, 107–110, 130, 131, 191
Self
  awareness, 135
  concept, 114, 125, 127
  sense organs, 21, 22, 24, 25
  sensory deprivation, 206
  integration, 123
  motor development, 212, 213, 217,
    225, 226